HEALING
ELEMENTS OF
DESIGN

CREATING TRANSCENDENT MEANING

A

HEALING ENVIRONMENTS/NIGHTWOOD

PUBLICATION

Design is Presence.

Design is Comfort.

Design is Relationship.

Contents

A moment of Maitri history is etched in my memory forever. Maitri, the fifteen-bed residential care facility for people living with AIDS, and Traci's first design job, was having its opening evening in San Francisco.

Two young gay men walked down the corridor. One of them took the other by the hand and led him into a small and lovingly designed bedroom. "This," he said, "is the room I would want to die in."

I've been trying to figure out why it is so difficult for me to tell people what Traci and I do. One reason, I think, is we are urging people in a secular society to embark on a sort of soul retrieval— to be cognizant of multiple levels of reality. I'm reminded of my favorite story about African bearers on a safari who, when asked why they were resting under a tree, responded, "We're waiting for our souls to catch up with our bodies."

The other reason is even more elusive. In all modesty, I believe we are trying to achieve something new (or rather something very old—something basic to ancient indigenous cultures). We are trying to teach people how to design from the heart (or soul), how to make their material world reflect spiritual realities, how to nourish themselves, their patients and loved ones with deeply healing environments.

Happily, there has been a shift in recent years from grey hospital walls to pretty pastels—from cold, sterile institutional environments to warm homelike healthcare settings. With astonishing results—the Barbara Karmanos Cancer Clinic in Michigan reports a 45% decrease in the need for pain medications since creating their healing environment.[1] But Traci and I hope to raise the bar even higher by asking the question, "Can healthcare environments nourish the soul as well as the body?"

I am reminded of my beloved mother-in-law, who spent her last three months in a prestigious teaching hospital. "Young man," she said to her attending resident in exasperation one day, "I'm more than a piece of meat!" A great deal of needless suffering occurs because we have tried to treat the patient's body without regard for his/her mind and soul. Hopefully, Lance Henderson, CFO of the San Francisco AIDS Foundation was correct when he credited Traci with setting a new standard in the field, by striving for the highest possible outcome—the healing of the whole patient.

So, when you wonder why there is a section on forgiveness in a book on design, we ask you to stretch your consciousness. Traci and I urge you to blur the line between interior and exterior, between the spiritual and the material, between mind, body and soul. In ancient Greek thought, *Kosmos* was the word for the universe—mind, body

---

1. Motoko Rich, "Healthy Hospital Designs," *Wall Street Journal* November 27, 2002

and spirit. There was no concept of the compartmentalization that exists today. Perhaps much of our suffering stems from our attempt to separate one from the other, when in reality no such separation exists. Modern psychoneuroimmunology teaches us that emotions are not, as previously thought, entirely localized in the brain, but rather spread throughout the body at the molecular level. This is the physiology of mind-body medicine.

But how does all this theory translate into actual healthcare settings? Let me give you a powerful example. Traci and I try to honor the spiritual depth of what a patient is going through. For example, when designing the corridor between the waiting room and treatment rooms in the West Cancer Clinic in Memphis, we hung a beautiful hand carved Indian door to symbolize the start of a transformative journey. Next to it we hung a soothing black and white photo with the title "comfort." The corridor itself was lined with more beautiful photos, all paired with healing words: compassion, grace, gratitude, forgiveness, hope, creativity, essence, light and finally transformation. Next to that final word stands a transcendent wooden sculpture of a set of wings, symbol of the Wings Cancer Foundation.

How much suffering might be eased if hospital emergency rooms offered soothing nature videos rather than contentious TV talk shows in their waiting rooms? What if anxious patients looking up found a frieze containing a loving kindness meditation? *May you be free from pain. May you be free from suffering. May your heart be at peace.*

Healing environments need not be expensive—they must, however, be inspired and intention-filled. The caregiver of a quad-replegic created this powerful healing environment: On the wall, at the foot of his bed, she had an artist paint a soaring eagle. Over his head, she constructed an arbor which enveloped him, and trained living plants to cover it. Finally she fulfilled his wish to see the moon by mounting a strategically-placed mirror. Her patient was so empowered by these healing intentions that he actually regained some movement. The healing environment enabled his spirit to soar.

We are asking you as individuals—as architects and designers, as patients and caregivers, to get in touch with the core of suffering—which lies as much in the soul or spirit as in the body. And to seek to soothe that suffering by bringing the exterior environment into alignment with the innermost needs of the patient. We are asking you to help us comfort the suffering by creating healing environments. Design from the heart. Design with the intention to heal. Create rooms which heal bodies, minds, and spirits. Create rooms where souls can rest in peace.

Bless you,

Kate

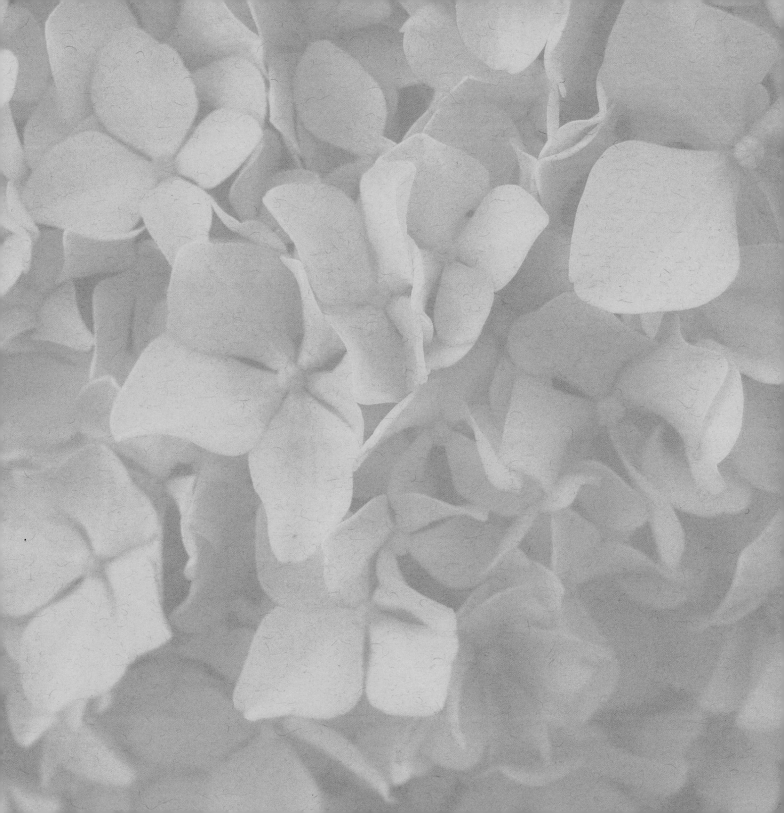

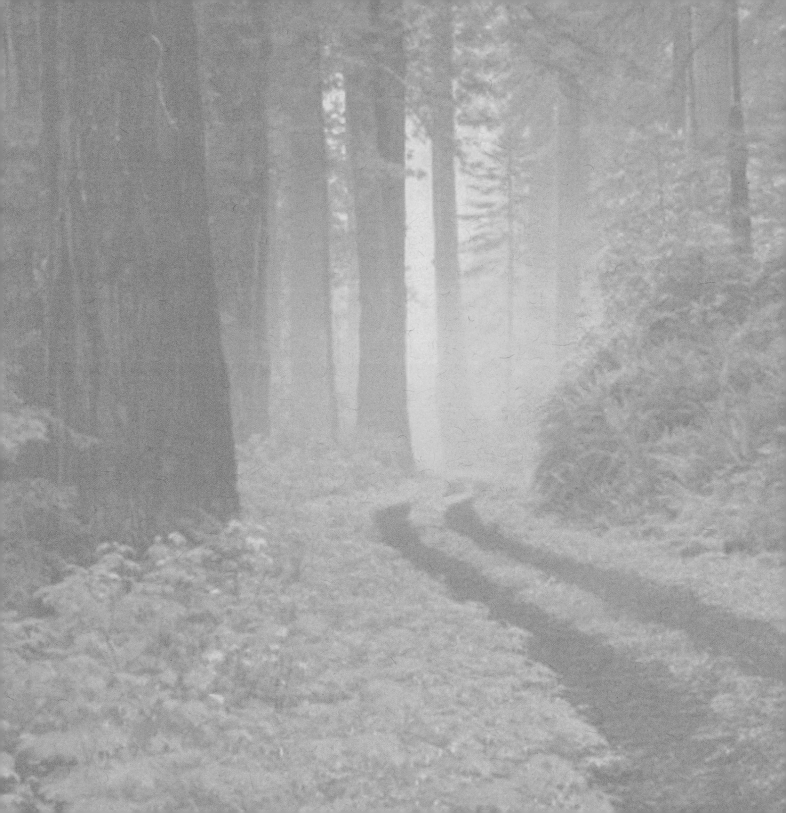

We are a small eleven-year-old non-profit organization dedicated to the relief of suffering of the seriously ill and to providing support to their families and caregivers with healing environments. How do we define a healing environment? We believe that it is one that offers sustenance to the soul and gives meaning to experience. A healing environment enables those who are suffering to transcend their pain by connecting to the universal and gives comfort through this connection.

There are three distinct areas in which we demonstrate our work philosophy: our resource center, our publications and our design work. We believe the transformative power of beauty, the arts and spirituality are tools that instill transcendent meaning into an environment and make it healing. It was Al Tarlov of the Kaiser Family Foundation who greatly inspired my partner Kate Strasburg when he said, ". . . If you want to change the world . . . start by creating a beautiful model." Healing Environments is our response to a void in the healthcare system that we hope to fill with our mission.

Our office is located in one of San Francisco's loveliest neighborhoods in a former antique store. In the front room visitors are welcomed into a home-like setting with comfortable couches and a beautiful array of meaningful art and objects. Bookshelves line the walls, filled to overflowing with books on art and design, spirituality, poetry and healing—as well as how to deal with illness, grief and loss. A large collection of video and audiotapes on these subjects are also available. We also have a room dedicated to the Jungian concept of sandtray. There are hundreds of evocative objects that fill the shelves in this room. The concept behind the sandtray is to empower the user to hand select objects that they are inherently drawn to and arrange them in a large container of sand. Metaphorically, the objects represent important symbols in that person's life. The sand-filled tray represents the subconscious mind.

Another area in which we demonstrate our mission is our journal, *A Light in the Mist: A Journal of Hope*. We send this publication several times a year to over 12,000 hospitals, hospices and individuals across the US and overseas. Currently, there are over 30 unique issues. Each issue has a different theme or topic, offering hope and comfort in the form of stories, poetry, and words of wisdom from writers, philosophers and theologians. *A Light in the Mist* reaches beyond the needs of the seriously ill, offering inspiration to all of us who struggle with life's challenges.

How might the healthcare setting support or compromise the wellbeing of a person, their family and friends? How do we

Excerpt from "The Temple of Amount" by Eliezer Shore, copyright © 1999 by
Eliezer Shore. Reprinted from *Parabola, The Magazine of Myth, Tradition, and the
Search for Meaning*, Vol. 24, No. 3, Fall 1999.

Excerpt from *Man's Search for Meaning* by Viktor E. Frankl, copyright © 1992
by Viktor E. Frankl. Used by permission of Beacon Press.

Excerpt from *The Book That Changed My Life* by Diane Olsen (editor), copyright © 2002 by Diane Osen. Used by permission of The Modern Library, an
imprint of Random House, Inc.

Excerpt from *The Art of Forgiveness, Lovingkindness, and Peace* by Jack Kornfield,
copyright © 2002 by Jack Kornfield. Used by permission of Bantam, an imprint of Random House, Inc.

Excerpt from *A Path with Heart* by Jack Kornfield, copyright © 1993 by Jack
Kornfield. Used by permission of Bantam, an imprint of Random House, Inc.

Excerpt from *100 Love Sonnets: Cien Sonetos de Amor* by Pablo Neruda, translated by Stephen Tapscott, copyright © 1959 and Fundacion Pablo Neruda,
copright © 1986 by the University of Texas Press. By permission of the University of Texas Press.

Text as submitted from p. 162 from *Small Wonder: Essays* by Barbara Kingsolver,
copyright © 2002 by Barbara Kingsolver. Reprinted by permission of Harper-
Collins Publishers.

Excerpt from pp. 190-1: "Our worst fear . . . liberates others." from *A Return to
Love* by Marianne Williamson, copyright © 1992 by Marianne Williamson.
Reprinted by permission of HarperCollins Publishers.

Excerpt from p. 119 from *The Soul's Religion* by Thomas Moore, copyright ©
2002 by Thomas Moore. Reprinted by permission of HarperCollins Publishers.

ACKNOWLEDGMENTS: Special thanks to Angela Castillo and Xenia Choubina
for their hard work, and to Sam Smidt for the transcendent beauty of his design.

transition from curing to healing? When technology, medicine, and our bodies fail, how can we support the spirit? How can the built environment support the world of healthcare, create a place of community and honor the individual?

When a person finds themselves in the role of the patient he often loses touch with the autonomy which has helped to shape his life. There is often a heightened emotional state and prolonged exposure to stress and alienation. A patient's perspective might be summarized by the following account in *Anatomy of an Illness* by Norman Cousins, former editor of the Saturday Review:

I know that during my own illness in 1964, my fellow patients at the hospital would talk about matters they would never discuss with their doctors. The psychology of the seriously ill put barriers between us and those who had the skill and the grace to minister to us. There was first of all the feeling of helplessness—a serious disease in itself. There was the subconscious fear of never being able to function normally again—and it produced a wall of separation between us and the world of open move-ment, open sounds, open expectations. The central question from Norman Cousins to be asked about hospitals or about doctors *is whether they inspire the patient with the confidence that he or she is in the right place. Whether they enable him to have trust in those who seek to heal him; in short, whether he has the expectation that good things will happen.*

In 1995 Healing Environments first encountered Maitri Hospice in San Francisco. This ten-year-old AIDS hospice was in the process of moving from an eight-bed Victorian to a newly refurbished building that would expand their services to become a licensable, fifteen-bed facility. Their model of care was built around the meaning of the Sanskrit word Maitri—compassionate friend-ship or loving kindness. It was evident in every person and their interactions with each other. There was a quality to the space that was hard to define: was it the people, the house they were in, the homemade food or the loving nursing staff?

The concern from the devoted staff and supporters of Maitri was that much of the soul would be lost if they were moved into a renovated parking garage. There was fear that what had taken years to create would be lost. What would be sacrificed in expanding the number of people served and moving to a licensable facility? As we began to work on the small meditation room the possibility arose for Healing Environments to assist with the whole design and installation of their interior environment. Our goal was to help preserve the integrity of the mission and to create a new home that would function better than the founding space.

With the talent of Joseph Chance of Kwan Henmi Architects, the structure would be infused with an abundance of natural light. The public areas and resident rooms would have large windows and a glass enclosed walkway between two courtyard gardens. The scale and proportion of the interior would feel welcoming. Courtesy of Healing Environments, each private resident room would have its own unique and practical furnishings that would provide character and charm. More importantly, there would be room to store personal belongings and both public and private spaces to be social in. The kitchen would be commercial-grade with a welcoming dining room. In the tradition of their former location, all meals would be homemade, nutritious and very appetizing.

It was shortly after the move into the new building that I walked past a resident's room, facing the interior courtyard. There was a young man lying in his bed and two women sitting near him. I asked if I could do anything for them and introduced myself as a volunteer who helped create the environment. The woman on the right stood up, approached me and thanked me for providing her son with a beautiful place to die. There are no other words to express why I believe so much in the power of creating healing environments.

I believe that physical transitions should be treated as a meaningful experience. Consider the path of the patient and caregiver. When we arrive in deep suffering our physical tolerance of all things shifts. Our own relationship to self and the world around us changes. In one of our earlier journals, we describe this place as *kairos*, the Greek word for spiritual time as opposed to *chronos*, chronological time.

There are opportunities to connect the individual to the space that they are in. As one approaches the building for the first time there is the inevitable apprehension of what one might encounter. Imagine the busy corner where several public train lines merge — constant rumbling, sometimes screeching sounds from the long cars as they busily traverse the city.

I would like to share with you part of the experience of Maitri: The experience begins with the exterior of the building. A core group of concerned staff and supporters suggested that the building be painted with bright colors that would enhance a formerly drab and dirty street corner. The colors suggest a connection back to their Asian roots with bright saffron and crimson red detail. When visitors approach the front doors they are greeted by a wooden arbor that resembles a Japanese Torii. The wood framing presents a human scale for the person entering the two story concrete building. From here, the path inside is reminiscent of a home — wood laminate flooring throughout the space, wooden handrails, lovely window coverings — touches that remind visitors that they are not in a traditional healthcare institution. There was a wall alongside the stairway that just seemed like a forgotten eyesore—so we asked a painter to create a mural resembling a Japanese screen painting. It features a tree at the ground level—that as one ascends the stairs becomes a landscape that shifts again when viewed from the top where it appears that you are on top of a mountain looking into a dreamy village below. There is an altar on the wall facing visitors at this point. We took Maitri's meaningful art and placed it in important places. In this case a colorful Mayumi Oda print of a goddess surrounded by an abundance of animals and vegetables. The small altar table is at once a greeting and a reminder of the important work that goes on daily. When a resident dies a candle is lit in his memory and his name is written in a small book. Those who wish to write in the book are invited to do so. It is a quiet and intimate experience.

To the right of the altar is the public living room which often reminds people of visiting a favorite relative or grandmother. It is cozy, nicely laid out with views into a well-tended garden. A focal point in this room is the donated Victorian wood fireplace mantel from a former neighbor. The detail and age of the piece immediately creates a sense of home. The dining area continues this philosophy and is a gathering place for some of the best cooked meals I have ever had. There are two long wood farm tables for ambulatory residents and staff. There is community created in sharing meals together. A beloved friend once said to me, "It takes just as long to create a good meal as it does a bad one." How often do you really enjoy the meal served in a healthcare facility?

Imagine the impact on a body that is starving for nutrition and that is met with nourishment for the soul as well as the senses. Each bedroom is a self-contained world. For some, it may be the nicest room they have had in life — for others, a reminder of how much their life has changed and that this is the end of their journey. We wanted to encourage each resident to decorate his room as he would like. Each piece of furniture is individualized and functional. The basics are all there including an armoire, a dresser, a bedside table with lamp, a chair (sometimes a sleeper style if a guest would like to stay), a TV, a clock/radio, and a view either towards the courtyard garden or out towards the urban environment.

I have learned so much from Maitri. Since our relationship began I have had the pleasure and honor of witnessing great love and spirit in those who have lived, worked and volunteered there. I have learned that we need to honor life until death arrives—that being alive is a gift and so many would wish for more time. That our relationships to one another and how we support those we love when they are suffering is essential to the quality of our lives and to the quality of our experience of death.

There is a quality to life that Maitri seeks to create for those whom they serve. Perhaps that is the quintessential difference between Maitri and standard institutions.

In offering to help we sought to soften the space, personalize it and make it feel like a home where the very real need to comfort the suffering is honored. I believe what we helped to create is a place of dignity and respect. If you are interested in learning more please contact Healing Environments at healingenvironments.org. For those interested in Maitri, please visit maitrisf.org.[2]

Bless you,.

Traci

---

2. This introduction was written in April 2005 when Traci spoke at the Architecture of Hospitals conference in Holland.

Healing
Elements of
Design

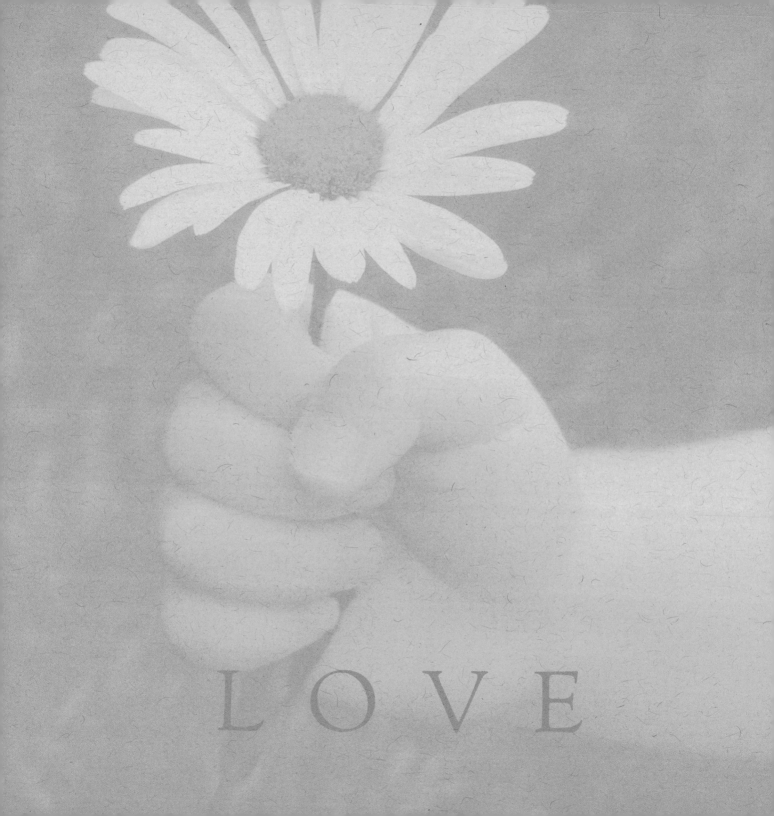

LOVE

Man's Search for Meaning

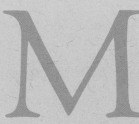

BY VIKTOR FRANKL

Salvation in a Concentration Camp

My mind still clung to the image of my wife. A thought crossed my mind: I didn't even know if she were still alive. I knew only one thing—which I have learned well by now: Love goes very far beyond the physical person of the beloved. It finds its deepest meaning in his spiritual being, his inner self. Whether or not he is actually present, whether or not he is still alive at all, cease somehow to be of importance.

I did not know whether my wife was alive, and I had no means of finding out (during all my prison life there was no outgoing or incoming mail); but at the moment it ceased to matter. There was no need for me to know: nothing could touch the strength of my love, my thoughts and the image of my beloved. Had I known then that my wife was dead, I think that I would still have given myself, undisturbed by that knowledge, to the contemplation of her image, and that my mental conversation with her would have been just as vivid and satisfying. "Set me like a seal upon thy heart, love is as strong as death."

A Path with Heart

ॐ

BY JACK KORNFIELD

MEDITATION ON FORGIVENESS

For most people forgiveness is a process. When you have been deeply wounded, the work of forgiveness can take years. It will go through many stages—grief, rage, sorrow, fear, and confusion—and in the end, if you let yourself feel the pain you carry, it will come as a relief, as a release for your heart. You will see that forgiveness is fundamentally for your own sake, a way to carry the pain of the past no longer. The fate of the person who harmed you, whether they be alive or dead, does not matter nearly as much as what you carry in your heart. And if the forgiveness is for yourself, for your own guilt, for the harm you've done to yourself or to another, the process is the same. You will come to realize that you can carry it no longer.

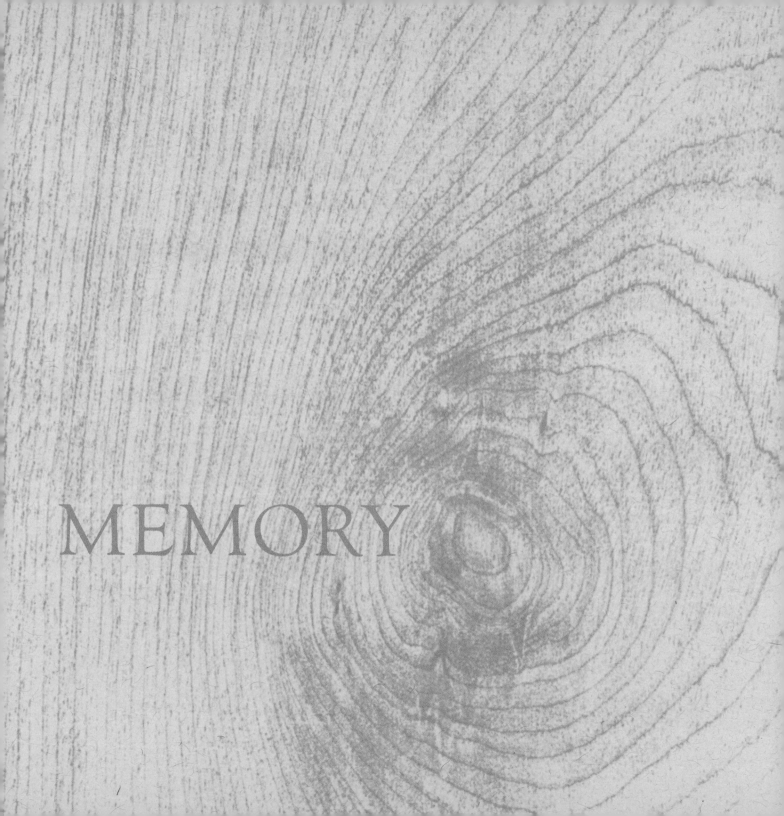

MEMORY

Small Wonder

୫

BY BARBARA KINGSOLVER

I am sitting on your lap, and you are crying. *Thank you, honey, thank you*, you keep saying, rocking back and forth as you hold me in the kitchen chair. I've brought you flowers: the sweet peas you must have spent all spring trying to grow, training them up the trellis in the yard. You had nothing to work with but abundant gray rains and the patience of a young wife at home with pots and pans and small children, trying to create just one beautiful thing, something to take you outside our tiny white clapboard house on East Main. I never noticed until all at once they burst through the trellis in a pink red purple dazzle. A finger-painting of colors humming against the blue air: I could think of nothing but to bring it to you. I climbed up the wooden trellis and picked the flowers. Every one. They are gone already, wilting in my hand as you hold me close in the potato-smelling kitchen, and your tears are damp in my hair but you never say a single thing but *Thank you*.

MEANING

There is nothing wrong in searching for happiness, but we use the term as if it were the ultimate in human striving. What gives far more comfort to the soul, I found in prison and in life, is something greater than happiness or unhappiness— and that is meaning. Meaning transfigures all.

—Sir Laurens van der Post

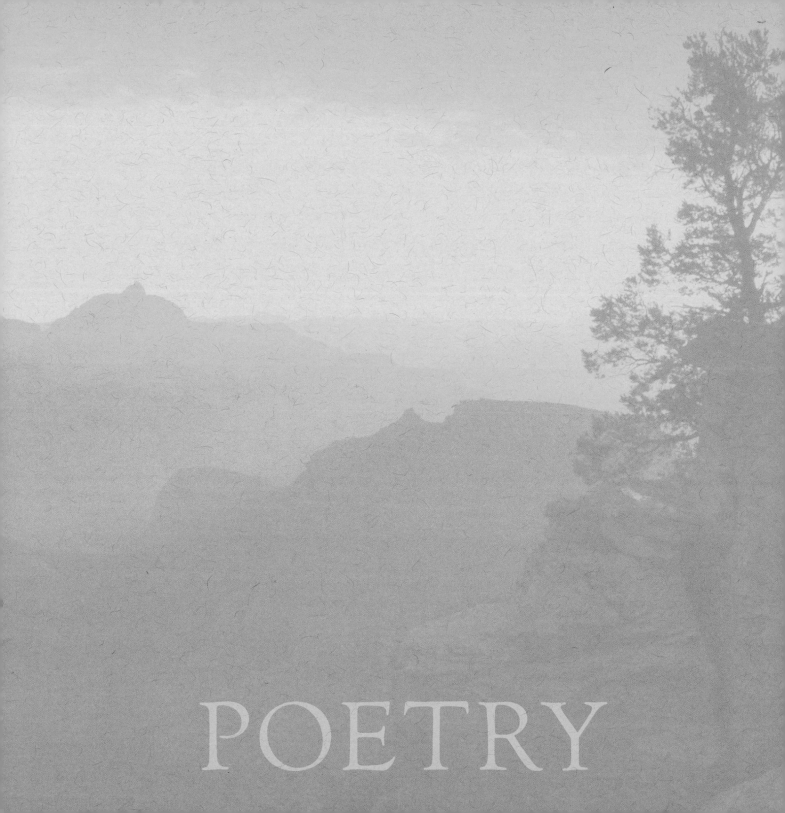

POETRY

Love Sonnet LXXXIX

ॐ

BY PABLO NERUDA

When I die, I want your hands on my eyes:
I want the light and the wheat of your beloved hands
to pass their freshness over me once more:
I want to feel the softness that changed my destiny.

I want you to live while I wait for you, asleep.
I want your ears still to hear the wind, I want you
to sniff the sea's aroma that we love together,
to continue to walk on the sand we walk on.

I want what I love to continue to live,
and you whom I love and sang above everything else
to continue to flourish, full-flowered:

so that you can reach everything my love directs you to,
so that my shadow can travel along in your hair,
so that everything can learn the reason for my song.

(EXCERPTED FROM *100 Love Sonnets*)

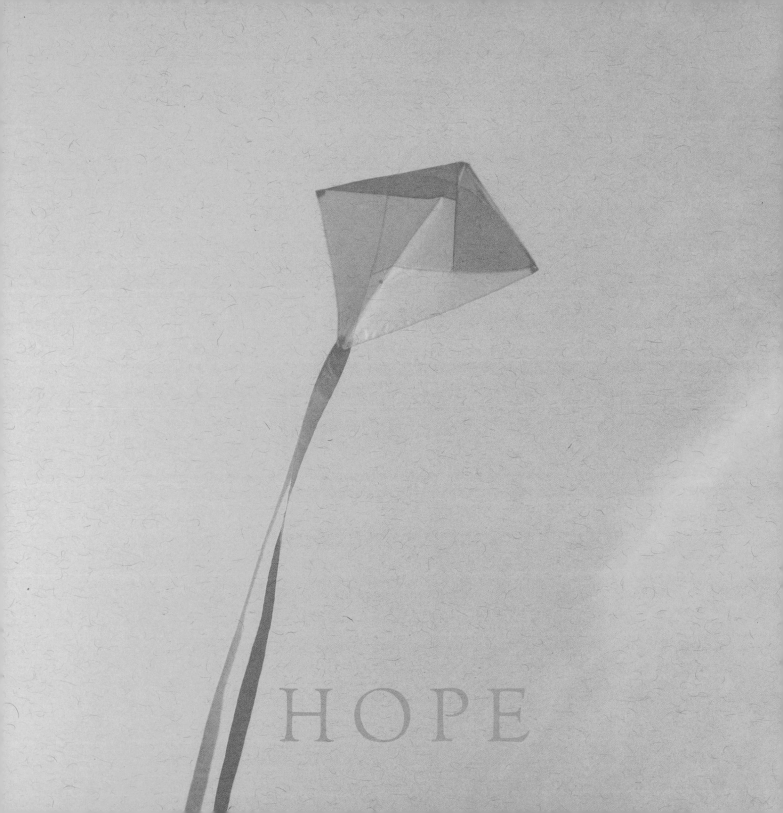

HOPE

Hope is the thing with feathers

That perches in the soul,

And sings the tune without the words,

And never stops at all.

—Emily Dickinson

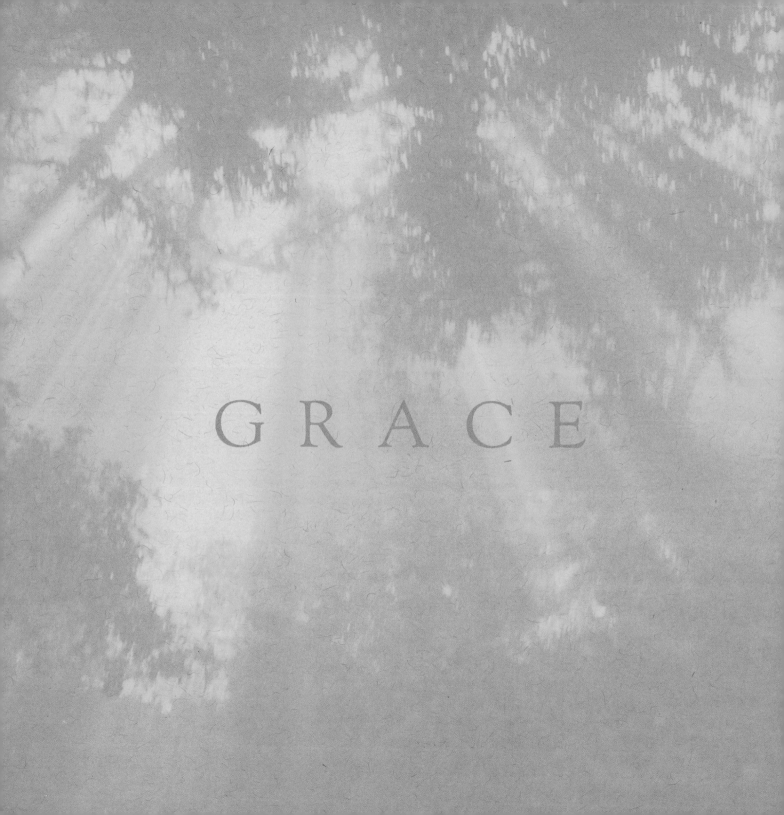

GRACE

Grace, Gratitude and Forgiveness

BY KATE STRASBURG

Grace has always meant mysterious and tender mercies to me. It has meant experiencing love when one feels least lovable, being healed in unexpected ways at unexpected times. Summed up in the words of Sister Corita Kent, "And there will be wonderful surprises." Perhaps to live life gracefully we need to ask for perpetual forgiveness, unending gratitude and the grace to experience both.

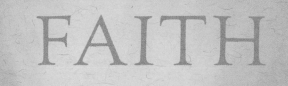

I said to my soul, be still,
and wait
without hope,

For hope would be hope
for the wrong
thing: wait without love

For love would be love
of the wrong
thing; there is yet faith

But the faith and the love
and the hope
are all in the waiting.

—T.S. Eliot

DESIGN

Healing Elements of Design

BY KATE STRASBURG AND TRACI TERAOKA

Two very attractive women walked into Hotel Monaco's Grande Café in San Francisco. Co-directors of Patient Support Services for a major cancer clinic in Memphis, Tennessee, they had come to the West Coast to gather ideas for how they might make their new facility a healing environment.

Under the leadership of Brenda Wiseman and Sandy Patterson, West Clinic Wings offers patients and their families the loving support that not only relieves suffering, but also promotes healing. "How can we extend our services to include the most healing environment possible?" they asked. This is our attempt to answer their question.

What can be done to ease the suffering of patients faced with a life-threatening diagnosis? What is a healing environment? A healing environment is one which connects the patient to that which is transcendent, and which brings comfort through that connection.

A patient who has been given a life-threatening diagnosis has had her world turned upside down. Unfortunately, clinical settings often reinforce this malaise with their sterility. How can architects and designers reverse this downward spiral?

First and foremost they must move beyond their formal training to a place of highest purpose and intention. They must realize it is within their power to alleviate suffering and this must be their primary goal. They may keep the following criteria in mind:

1. SEEK TO GROUND THE PATIENT IN THE WORLD AT LARGE.

Use natural materials such as beautiful woods, stone, and slate, to connect the patient to the outside world.

Introduce nature itself in the form of living plants, running water, and beautiful orchids.

Incorporate natural lighting and provide access to fresh air through skylights, courtyards, and atriums.

❧ Appeal to all five senses through light, color, texture, music, comfort foods, and natural light scent. (A hospital in Minnesota has a hundred-track sound system which replicates the sounds of a country river.)

❧ Include items with age (antiques) and hand-crafted artifacts to place patients in a larger context of time. Comfort patients with the essence of home: comfortable furniture, coffee, and access to kitchens.

2. Offer the option of transcendence. (Especially important for the patient whose life is threatened and for his or her loved ones.)

❧ Create special and easily accessible places for prayer and meditation.

❧ Keep a sense of mystery, of that which we cannot know. There is comfort in the concept that man is not the measure of all things.

❧ Incorporate icons and symbols of transcendence. Avoid the denominational and seek the universal.

(Better a chapel with a fountain and orchids than one with symbols of eight belief systems.)

🌿 Attempt through symbols to transcend both time and space.

3. COUNTERACT THE SENSE OF DISEMPOWERMENT AND LOSS OF IDENTITY WHICH OFTEN ACCOMPANIES SERIOUS ILLNESS.

🌿 Where possible offer choice (bed linens? bed surrounds? art from an art cart for bedroom walls?).

🌿 Encourage self-expression by having art studios, sandtray rooms, and video rooms (for creating family heirlooms).

🌿 Incorporate in each patient's room a means of expressing and celebrating his individuality. (A locked display case? A frame on the door for a photograph and bio?)

🌿 Offer easily accessible patient libraries for medical information regarding treatment.

🌿 Replace the ubiquitous TV with a VCR and consider individual CD players with earphones.

4. ATTEMPT TO PLACE THE PATIENT'S EXPERIENCE IN A CONTEXT THAT MAY GIVE IT MEANING, THEREBY REDUCING SUFFERING.

❧ Where possible offer healing, as opposed to merely decorative art. What is healing art? Healing art is art which relates to the depth of the patient's experience, rather than glossing over it.

❧ Consider the healing power of literature. Incorporate inspiring quotes and poetry.

❧ Avoid minimalism and replace it with a rich layering of detail. When facing death, what may be excellent design feels cold and impersonal. Avoid the color grey.

5. CONSIDER THE WELL-BEING OF THE PATIENT, THE FAMILY AND THE MEDICAL STAFF TO BE INSEPARABLE. (THEY FORM A TRIUMVIRATE AND EACH AFFECTS THE OTHER.)

❧ Offer all three populations means of self-expression, avenues for grieving and inspiration for healing.

❧ Make waiting rooms and examining rooms as healing as individual patient rooms.

MEDITATION

The Art of Forgiveness,
Lovingkindness, and Peace

BY JACK KORNFIELD

May I and all beings
be free from pain and sorrow.
May I and all beings
be held in compassion.
May I and all beings
be reconciled.
May I and all beings
be at peace.

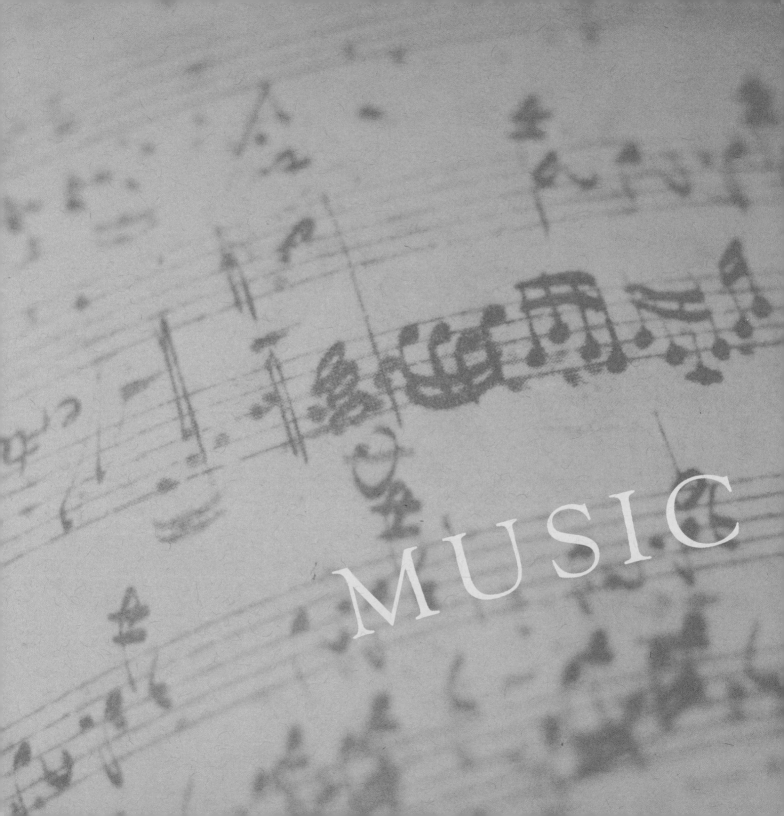

Music is My Medicine

✦

BY MAUREEN MCCARTHY DRAPER

We go to music for so many things. Joyful, sad, playful, lonely—music has the power to arouse our passion or to still it, to validate and enhance a mood or to change it. But whether we want to deepen or lighten our spirit, when music gives form to feeling it relieves us of carrying the full burden inside. And with expression comes a certain freedom and sense of being more in harmony with ourselves. Paradoxically, as we listen to music we are also listening to ourselves. The music is a bridge between our inarticulate world of thought and sensation and the outer world.

All the elements of music combine to work their magic. A melody or harmony may suddenly move us to tears—or elation. Slow rhythms tend to relax and steady, faster rhythms to increase pulse and breath rate. If we're in physical or emotional pain, music can take us out of ourselves, reminding us there is another reality of beauty and sensuous pleasure. Outer harmony helps restore inner harmony. And we may never need this more than when we are hospitalized for an accident or illness.

DECEMBER 28, 2002

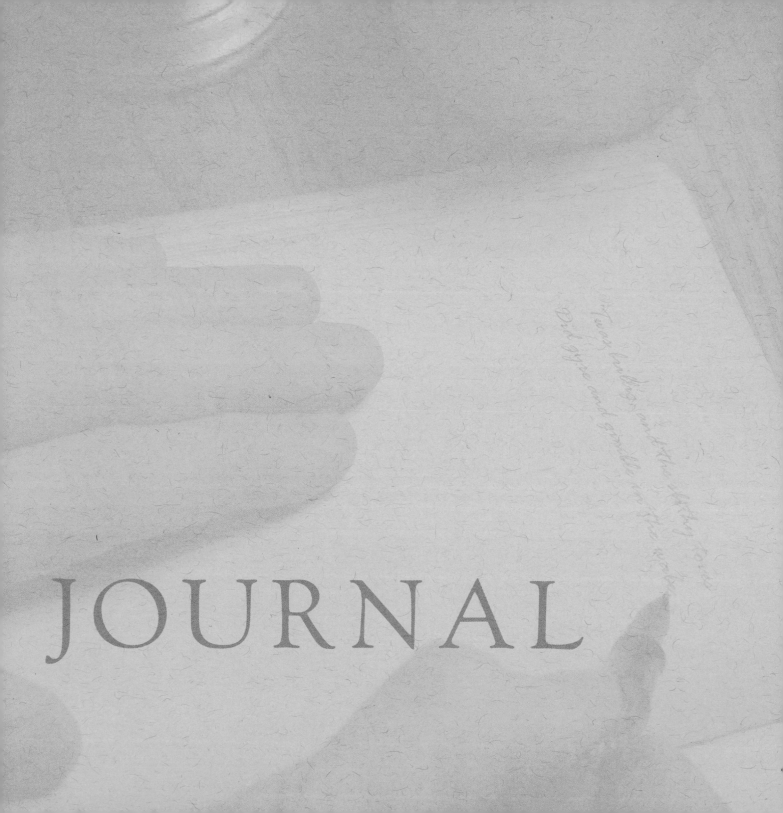

JOURNAL

Into the Well: Keeping a Journal with Ira Progoff

≈

BY DOREE ALLEN

We are engaged in entering the well of our life and in reaching as deeply into its sources as we can. —Ira Progoff

I suspect that, like me, many of you have lingered over the "blank book" section of your favorite art or stationery store, contemplating the perfect journal—the one bound simply in rice paper, perhaps, that will finally inspire your personal practice of writing. Although journaling has had a renaissance of sorts in the past few years, keeping a diary is one of the oldest methods of self-exploration, and while we may all have different notions of what constitutes a diary or journal, most of us have sought the silent, spacious counsel of its pages at one time or another.

Before you buy that new blank book, though, I would urge you to consider a different approach to keeping a journal; one that combines what we typically think of as keeping a diary with an innovative, more structured format known as the *Intensive Journal Process*.

Drawing on both Jungian principles and depth psychology, it is a method developed by the psychologist Ira Progoff and considered by Joseph Campbell "one of the great inventions of our time."

I first became aware of the *Intensive Journal Process* from an invitation I received to attend one of the many workshops that are offered throughout the country. Included in the literature about the program was an interview with Dr. Progoff that immediately intrigued me, especially by what he had to say about the benefits of working with the process and the ways it differed from a traditional approach to keeping a journal:

It helps us to see the movement of our life history as a whole, from the vantage point of the present moment. It also helps us to position ourselves between the past and the future so we can support the unfoldment of new potentials in our life…. When journal keeping is not related to the larger development of one's life as a whole, it lacks a sustaining principle. Often it is resorted to when a person has a particular goal in mind, such as finding a new career path or establishing a specific love relationship, but when the goal is achieved the journal falls into disuse and the continuity of the life context as a whole is lost. No overall integration or self-exploration results…. Working with the process enriches our inner life immea-

surably, helping us to stay in touch with that underlying reality which is
our personal source of meaning and strength.

Progoff's method asks us to look particularly at four dimensions of our experience: Life/Time, Dialogue, Depth and Meaning, and within these categories helps us to find the thread of continuity that is moving throughout our life. It reminds us of our life's stepping-stones, our dreams and mentors, and of those intersections where roads taken and not taken may be reassessed and revisited. And whether you attend a workshop, as I did, where someone leads you through the various exercises or you use Dr. Progoff's book, *At a Journal Workshop*, as a guide, you will be given a gentle framework for evoking new ideas and opening contexts of understanding. For in the reciprocal movement between past and present is the gift of perspective—something we all need at our century's turn.

At the heart of the Journal Workshops is the metaphor of the well connected to an underground stream. The invitation Progoff extends to us is to reach as deeply into the sources of our well as we can, so that in the depths we may someday take flight.

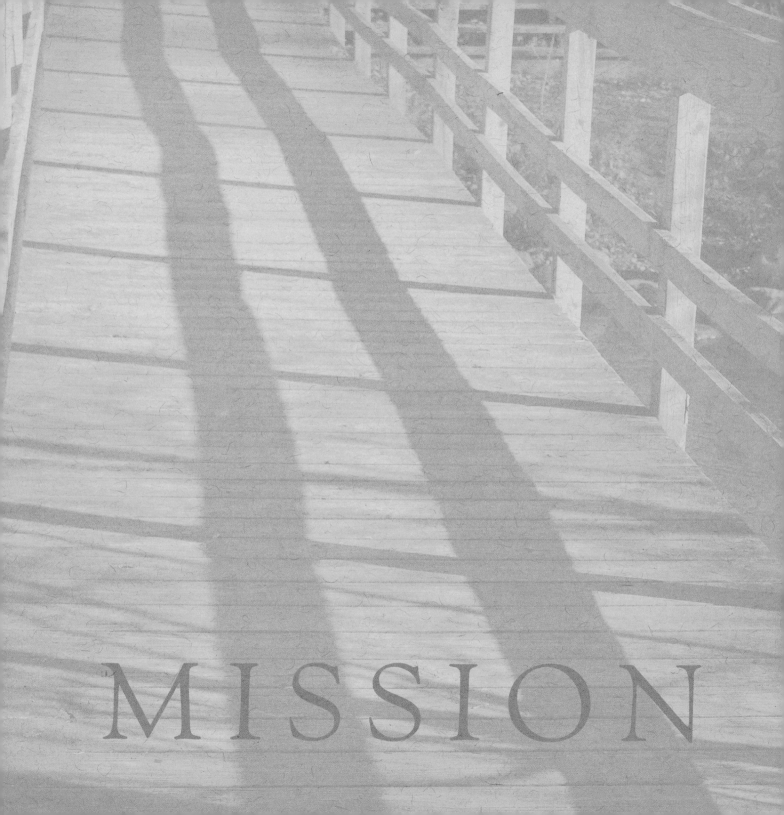

MISSION

A Return to Love

BY MARIANNE WILLIAMSON

Our worst fear is not that we are inadequate, our deepest fear is that we are powerful beyond measure. It is our light, not our darkness that most frightens us. We ask ourselves, "Who am I to be brilliant, gorgeous, talented and fabulous?" Actually who are you not to be? You are a child of God; your playing small doesn't serve the world. There is nothing enlightened about shrinking so that other people won't feel insecure around you. We were born to make manifest the glory of God within us. It is not just in some of us, it is in everyone and as we let our own light shine we unconsciously give other people permission to do the same. As we are liberated from our own fear our presence automatically liberates others.

WORK

Work is Love Made Visible

BY KAHLIL GIBRAN

And what is it to work with love?

It is to weave the cloth with threads drawn from your heart, even as if your beloved were to wear that cloth.

It is to build a house with affection, even as if your beloved were to dwell in that house.

It is to sow seeds with tenderness and reap the harvest with joy, even as if your beloved were to eat the fruit.

It is to charge all things you fashion with a breath of your own spirit,

And to know that all the blessed dead are standing about you and watching.

...

Work is love made visible.

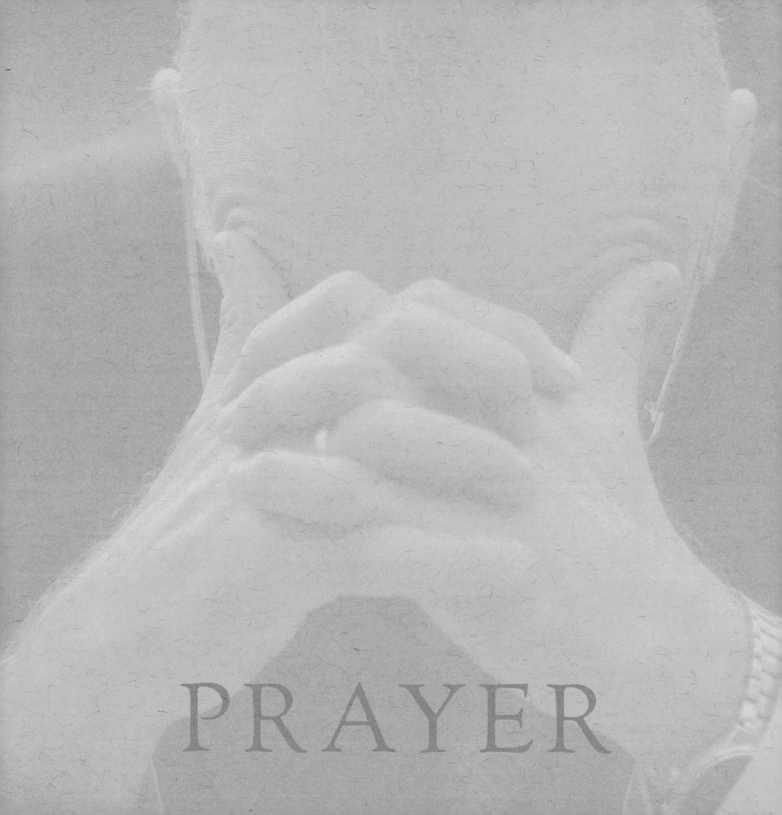
PRAYER

The fruit of silence is prayer

The fruit of prayer is faith

The fruit of faith is love

The fruit of love is service

The fruit of service is peace

—MOTHER TERESA

COMPASSION

On the Nature of Compassion

BY KATE STRASBURG

"I am sorry to have to hurt you," the doctor said. My eyes welled up with tears. Not because of the pain. Because of the compassion. In ten years of intrusive tests for my condition, no one had ever acknowledged my pain.

All of the world's greatest spiritual traditions stress the importance of compassion. From the Latin *cum passio*—meaning "with suffering"—compassion is the gift of "being with one who is suffering." For nothing increases another's suffering more than a sense of isolation; a sense of being alone with one's pain.

What is the path to compassion?

First and foremost, in order to feel compassion for others, we must feel compassion for ourselves. To connect with the pain of others, we must have connected with our own pain. In order to do so, one must let go of fear and also of judgement. For compassion and judgement cannot go hand in hand.

Secondly, and this is extremely difficult in Western society, we must let go of the need to "fix" things. One of the greatest barriers to a sense of compassion is Western arrogance. A hard lesson of the AIDS epidemic has been that for the first time in recent history, Western medicine has been faced with human suffering on an overwhelming scale. Suffering for which there is no cure. Suffering which we cannot "fix." Americans have been forced to confront their fear of death, their denial of death, their tendency to see death as defeat.

We have been forced to discover a new reality—the reality of transcendence. The reality that one can be "healed" without being "cured." The reality that quality of life may be more important than quantity. The mystery that tragedy may beget epiphany, and that a spiritual awakening may be born from an epic epidemic.

But how can one rest in the face of death, day after day, without being numbed by the pain? We secular Americans have tended to stress self-reliance and stoicism. These will not serve us for the long haul. Those of us who do not have spiritual traditions will have to learn to look deep within. We will need to draw on our higher selves, on the universe if not on a deity, to renew ourselves in our commitment to compassion. We will need to explore tools of renewal, such as meditation, to be refreshed and reborn daily. For as a Japanese sage once said: "A clear wind can blow ten thousand miles."

So then, let us create a circle of compassion. For ourselves. For our loved ones. For all those struggling with life-threatening illness. For their caregivers. For their medical personnel. Let us, like Maitri, form a community of compassion. Let no one suffer alone.

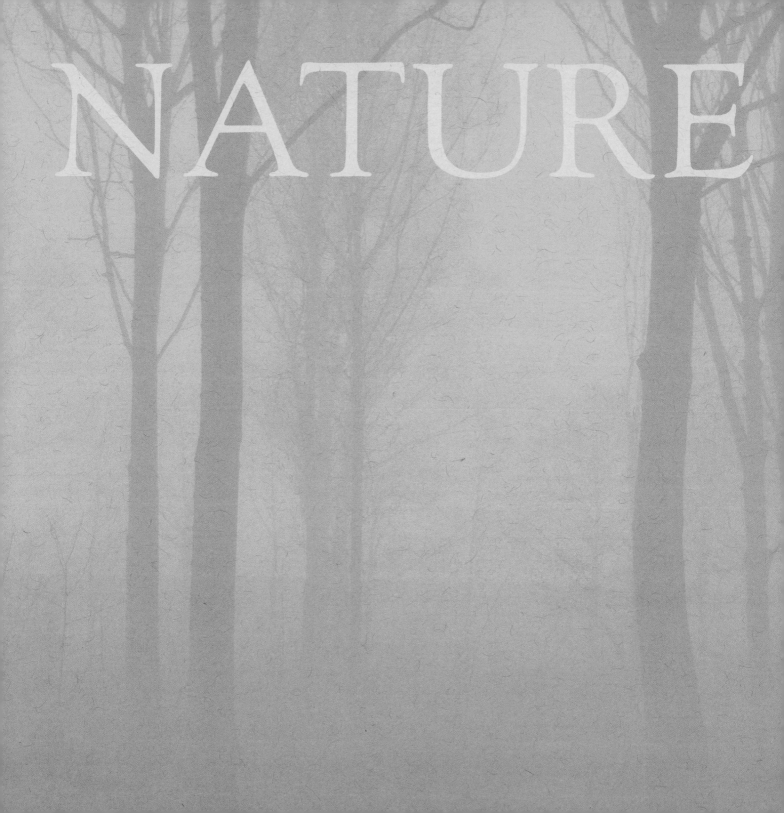

The Peace of Wild Things

BY WENDELL BERRY

When despair for the world grows in me
and I wake in the night at the least sound
in fear of what my life and my children's lives may be,
I go and lie down where the wood drake
rests his beauty on the water, and the great heron feeds.
I come into the peace of wild things
who do not tax their lives with forethought
of grief. I come into the presence of still water.
And I feel above me the day-blind stars
waiting with their light. For a time
I rest in the grace of the world, and am free.

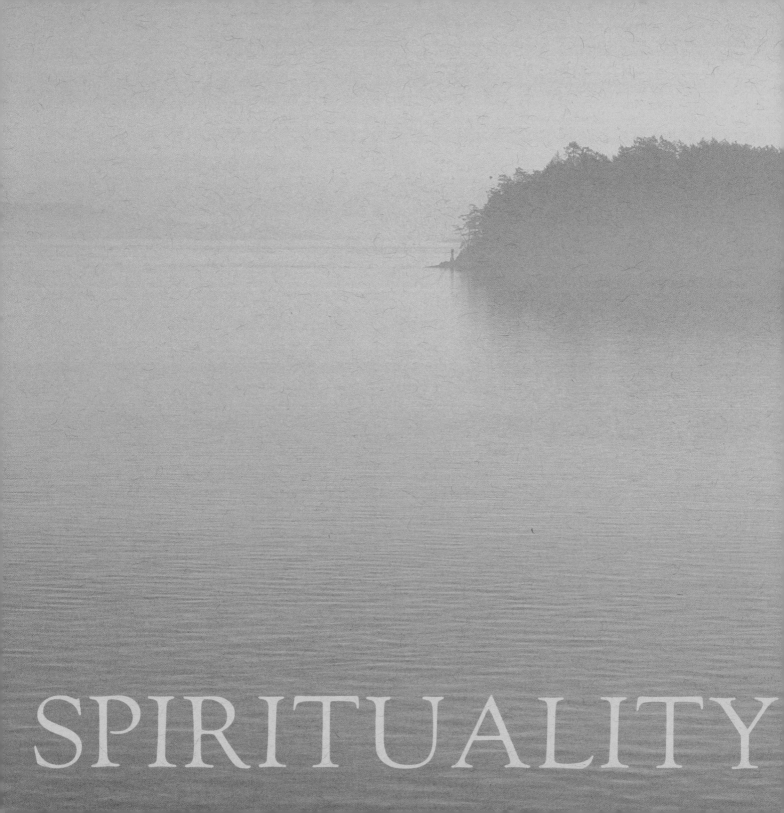

SPIRITUALITY

The Soul's Religion

❦

BY THOMAS MOORE

The Soul's Religion

The unpleasant sensation of falling apart need not be literally negative. It can open us up to receive the creative impulses of the spirit and take another step toward what fate has in store for us. Let's look even more closely now at ordeals, at the initiatory aspect of falling apart. This is one way spirit and soul come together. The emotional struggle, engaged but not necessarily "won," affects the soul profoundly and allows us to have a larger view of life and its mysteries. Initiations—it seems we're always in one or another—pulverize those parts of us that are rigid and break up self-protective explanations and understandings. The suffering involved allows something infinitely large to penetrate, and simple pain turns into ordeal, trial, and initiation. The passages of the soul give birth to the spirit.

WRITING

The Book That Changed My Life

ॐ

EDITED BY DIANE OLSEN

What transforms the merely sad into
something tragic—and therefore
beautiful, and therefore saving, and
therefore, in some odd way, joyful—is
the telling of the story. It's what
makes us human beings.

—James Carroll

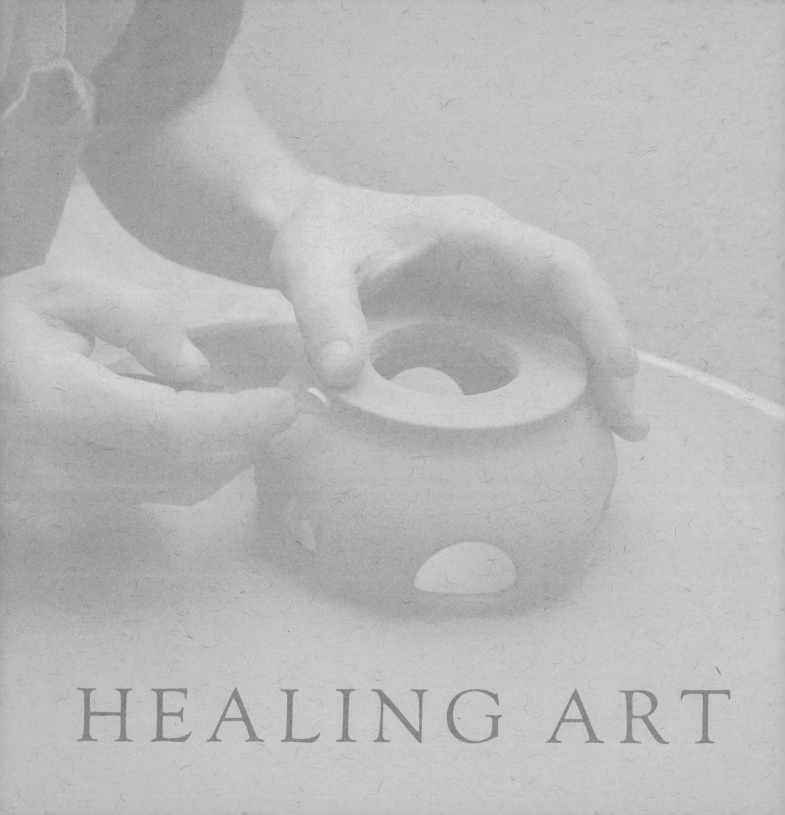

HEALING ART

Healing Art

⁊⁊

BY KATE STRASBURG

Our space at Healing Environments is filled with healing art. What do we mean by "healing" art? Healing art is art which enables the viewer to transcend his pain (whether emotional or physical) by connecting him to a sense of the universal. This connection is both grounding and comforting. It presents a larger context in which the viewer feels supported and sustained.

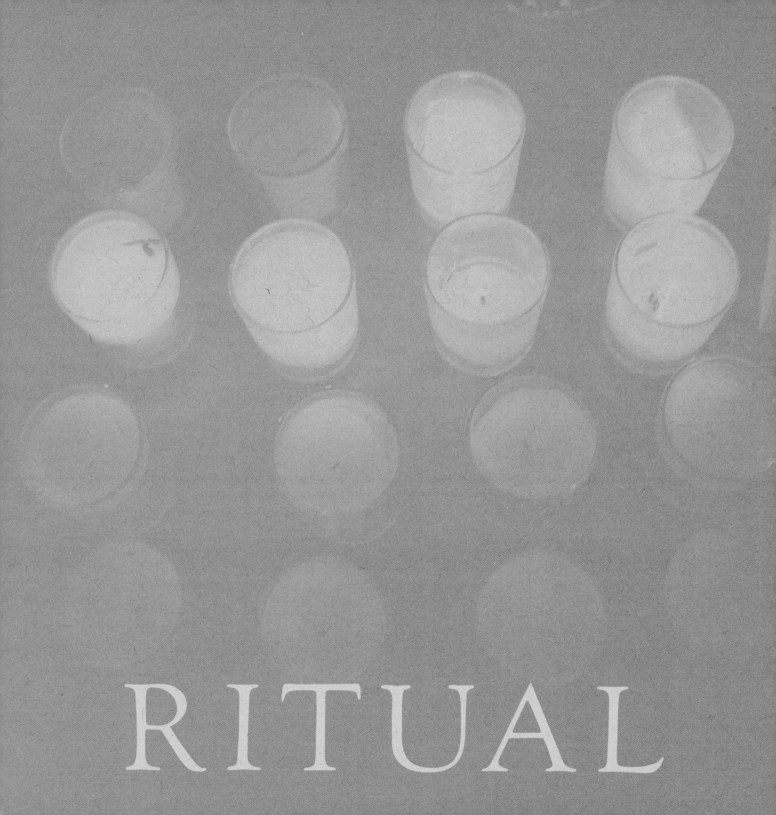

RITUAL

The Power of Ritual

BY KATE STRASBURG

To a large extent, modern man has lost the power of ritual. In his efforts to be rational, he has forsaken the mystery of the universe. Many of us have left organized religion behind, creating a void of meaning. As the century ends and we face the new millennium in fear and uncertainty, more and more of us are exploring ancient ways and forgotten wisdom to replace what we have lost. The twentieth century, born in arrogance and boundless optimism, humbled us with the limits of our knowledge. Let us use our newfound humility to ask for guidance, to seek for solutions larger than science, deeper than materialism. Let us create personal rituals that connect us to our common humanity, which infuse our struggles with meaning, which frame our search for solutions. Let us reopen to the mystery of existence.

CREATIVITY

There is a vitality, a life force, an energy, a quickening that is translated through you into action. And because there is only one of you in all time, this expression is unique. And if you block it, it will never exist through any other medium... The world will not have it. It is not your business to determine how good it is, nor how valuable, nor how it compares with other expressions. It is your business to keep it yours clearly and directly, to keep the channel open.

—Martha Graham

SYMBOLS

The Temple of Amount

&

BY ELIEZER SHORE

Every symbol carries some inner meaning, whether simple or complex. In all cases, a symbol is an object whose content is greater than its form, for with just a few lines or gestures it conveys a message that would otherwise require many words. But precisely because of this meager form, because their meaning is not overt, symbols demand that the viewer reconstruct the original message within himself. As such, they are vehicles for inner transformation, and are among the primary tools of the religious life, which seeks to convey truths that are altogether beyond words. Symbols are points of contemplation, for only by dwelling upon them are their contents revealed. And the more one contemplates them, the more meaningful they become. Furthermore, religious symbols, whose subject is the infinite, have the potential to convey an infinity of meaning.

EXCERPTED FROM *Parabola*, FALL 1999

INTENTION

Maitri Revisited

BY TRACI TERAOKA

Bless the soul that lives herein...
Go confidently in the direction of your dreams.
Act as though it were impossible to fail.
　　　　　　　—Dorothea Brandt

As I sit down to write an update about our design work in San Francisco, I am reminded of this quotation. As co-directors of Healing Environments, Kate and I have encountered many people and situations that have affected our work—as we continue to grow, our priorities must adjust to our needs—it is in trying to meet our mission statement that I feel most humble. The work that we seek to create at Healing Environments might puzzle some, inspire others, and hopefully, at its most powerful and sincere effort, comfort many.

MAITRI: RESIDENTIAL CARE FOR
PEOPLE LIVING WITH AIDS
SAN FRANCISCO, CALIFORNIA

Maitri is completely occupied. Fifteen bedrooms are now micro-
cosms to their inhabitants. At press time, six residents will have
passed away since Maitri opened its doors in November.[3] I drop by
weekly to check on things and to stay connected to them.

I believe we breathe life into our work by maintaining a relationship with it. Almost every time I visit, I am bewildered by the
amount of work that can still be done. More art. More funky,
handmade accoutrements. New "this" and different "that." I have
to remind myself that no project is ever completely finished. Life as
process. Design as process.

I think one of the most troublesome aspects of renovation and
expansion projects is the realization that what has taken years to
create will be lost. It came in different stages at Maitri—first with the
staff move to the new address, secondly when the residents moved
in. The "flow" was different. Walking through the halls and living
rooms felt unfamiliar. There was a despair at times that the "soul"
was lost. What had they sacrificed to move from a home to a home-
like facility?

I consulted with a friend whom I have known for years—who has
often lent wisdom and kind words during hard times—I explained

---

3. This article was written in 1995.

the sense of sadness and abandonment I felt inhabiting the hospice, and she passed on these words: "...let them know it is okay to feel grief and loss over the move. The people that are making the transition were initially drawn there for a reason. There is a sense of loss—the love and work they have put into the original will be missed. More importantly, the people at the core (the executive director and core staff) need to create a new vision and fan the flames of that vision. The group wants to be on board—they just don't have a new vision to hold on to yet."

I have become more involved in the transition of moving into a new space. We all know it is difficult and exciting, but we try to settle in as if it were routine. Consider this as an opportunity: What if we consider moving as an opportunity to refuel our intentions—to name what is important to us and place that knowledge on every doorway, every window, every room? In Japan my ex-husband Rick and I witnessed a new taxi being blessed at a temple for wealth and prosperity. At the time we thought it was unusual and a bit funny, but it makes a lot of sense to me now. Be deliberate about your intentions—make it happen.

A special thanks to the people that live and work at Maitri for allowing me to continue to learn from their home. It is the most heartfelt education that I have ever received.

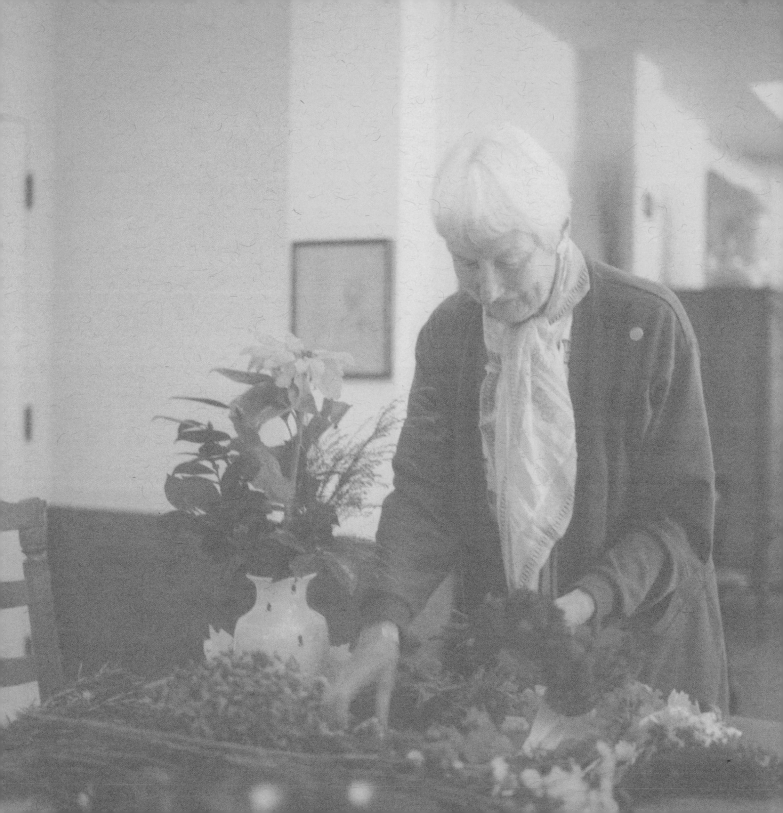

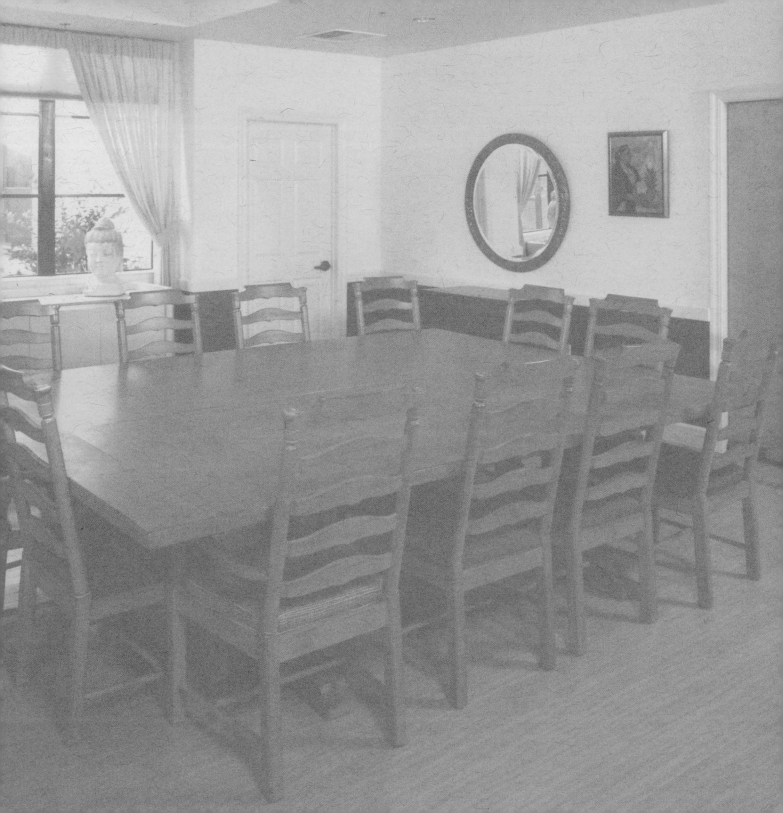

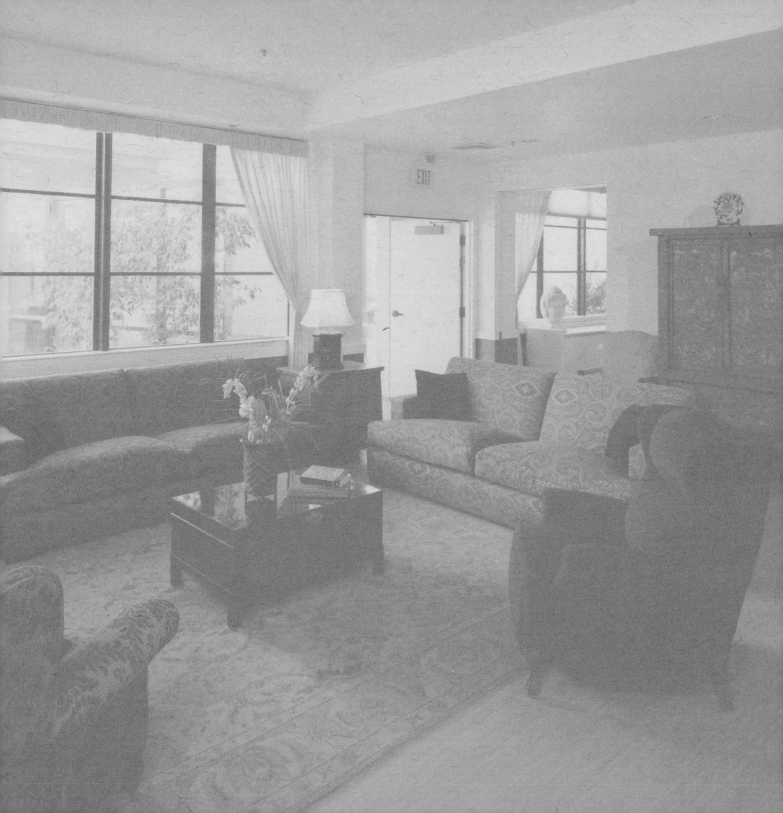

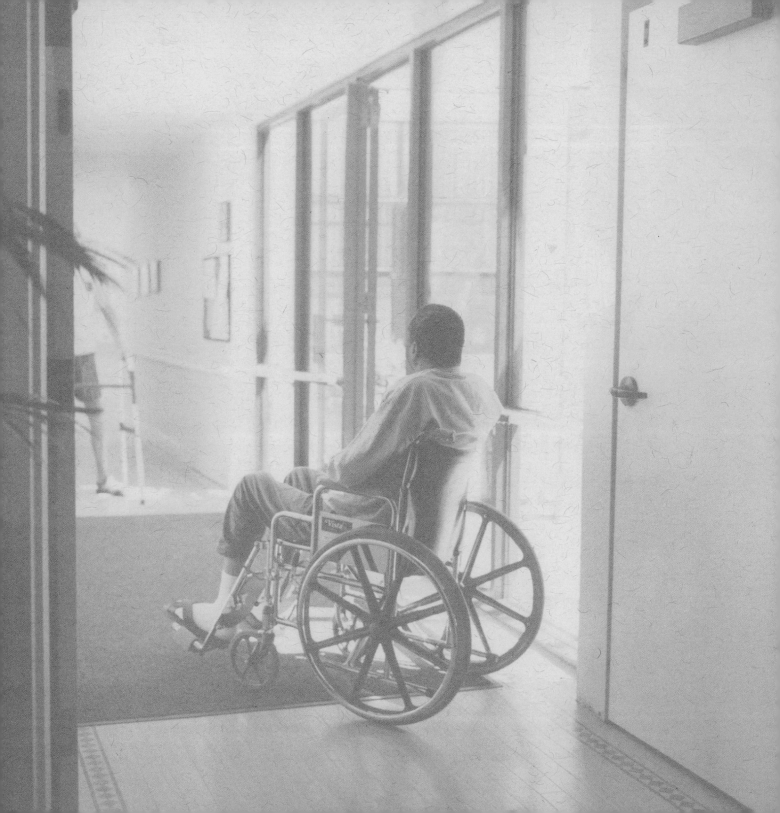

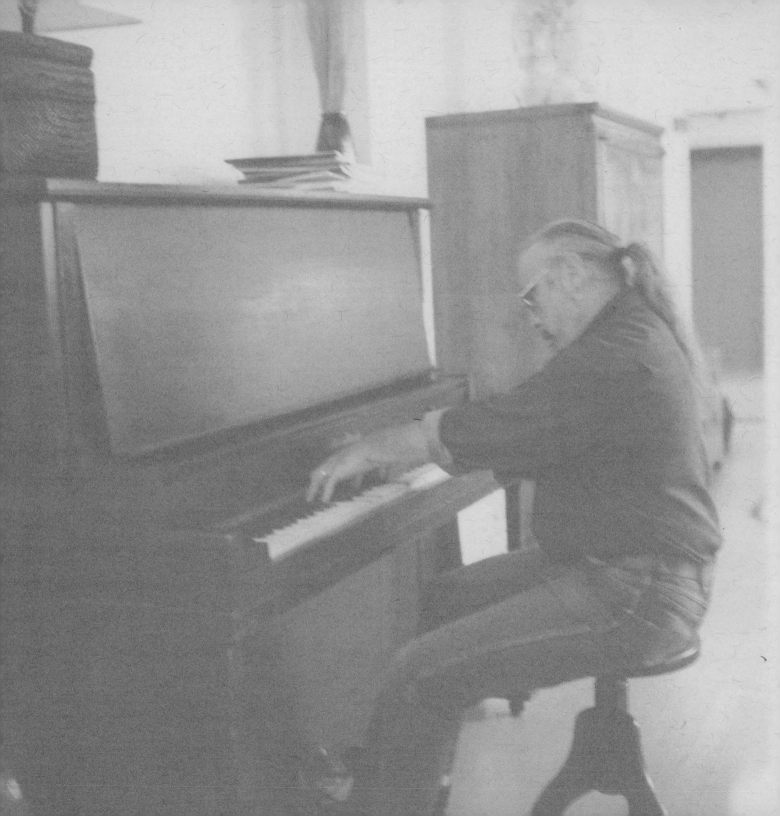

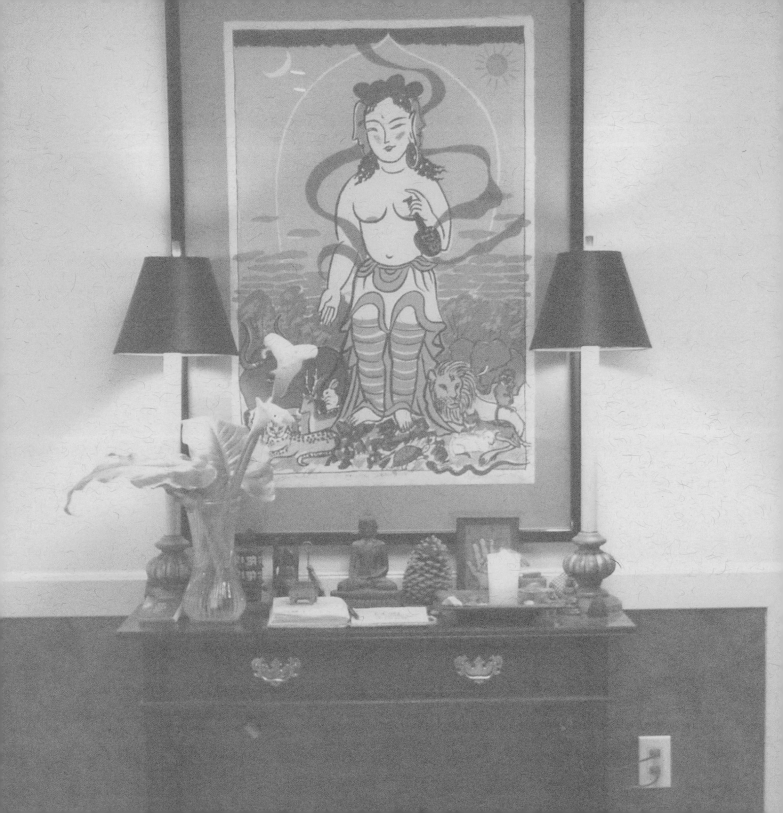

DESIGN

Giving Form to your Vision

⌘

BY KATE STRASBURG

One November Traci and I were invited to address the Symposium on Healthcare Design in San Francisco. A great deal of good arose from this conference, but our favorite part of the presentation was an experiential exercise that we led. Our goal was to help our audience learn to design from "the inside out." By asking them to identify with a patient's deepest needs, we hoped to help them better address those needs.

We have included the exercise in this book in the hopes that it may help other architects and designers, as well as patients, their families and caregivers. Like all exercises which explore our deepest truths, it can only bring us closer to our most essential selves. And in sharing those truths it can only bring us closer to one another.

For this exercise, image it is
you who is seriously ill.

EXERCISE

What can you do to comfort yourself?
What healing environment can you create?
How can you make it a haven? How can you
imbue it with comfort? What soothing sense
of order, what personal expression will ground
you? How can you expand time by infusing it
with memory, with a sense of meaning? How
can you celebrate your life, your identity?

What personal icons or symbols can serve as touchstones? What rituals can you create to overcome both time and distance, to transcend the limitations your illness has placed on you? How can you use your physical surroundings to return you to your essence? How can this illness become your key to transformation? How can it lead you into the light?

HEALING HOME

The Healing Home

෨

BY KATE STRASBURG

In this world of increasing stress and complexity all of us need a haven, a healing environment, a healing home. As the information age hurls us into cyberspace, how can we remain grounded, centered, secure? The answer is not to acquire more, but rather to seek more meaning in what we acquire. To pause and look inward and—as African bearers resting beside the trail once said—"Wait for our souls to catch up with our bodies."

I first met Traci, my co-director at Healing Environments, when I was furnishing a ski condo I had recently found. At the time, Traci was managing an antique store and I, recently divorced, was trying to create a sense of stability in the midst of chaos. How could I give my children a sense of continuity in their changing world? In a culture which values what is new over what is old, how could I give them both a sense of time and place that would subtly convey transcendence and enduring values?

Surprisingly, with Traci's help, I discovered some things which both grounded me in who I was and soothed the children by the expression of that reality. As a former French teacher and Catholic convert, I was stunned to find a set of antique leather bound books from a convent in the old French walled city of Carcasonne in her shop on a small California suburban street. As I leafed through the works of St. John of the Cross and St. Teresa of Avila, small cards belonging to novitiates over a hundred years ago fell from their pages. I was both transported in time and space to a reality larger than my personal odyssey.

Having lived both on the East Coast and in France, I have often thought how we in America, especially in the West, suffer from a lack of history. There is something soothing about being cradled in a context larger than our own. Sleeping in a two-hundred-year-old house in Massachusetts or a two-hundred-year-old apartment in Paris, one cannot help but feel supported by the experience of generations of predecessors.

The average American moves five times in a lifetime, often thousands of miles away from family and community. How can we create a context for ourselves which will nourish us in times of adversity? The answer is to journey inward on a journey of self-discovery and, at the same time, to place that rediscovered self in a larger supportive framework. The homes which we create for ourselves can become representative of both who we are and what supports us—physical symbols of both the inner self and the outer universe.

When visitors tour our showcase of ideas in San Francisco, almost without exception they speak of the special energy which they experience—the deep sense of peace which supports and renews them. Let me try to share with you the component parts of this—the healing elements of design.

ANTIQUES

Age

BY KATE STRASBURG

One way that design can place us in a larger context is through the medium of age. I came to a love of antiques late in life. What something with age does for us is to place our concerns in a proper context. The patina of a well-worn piece of wood speaks of crises weathered and survived. Those of us lucky enough to have family heirlooms know of what I speak. Eating holiday meals at a table that has seen decades of the same gives a sense of security and containment. If we have no such heritage, we may borrow it by filling our lives with things that have brought others comfort in the past. Furniture need not be costly to be reassuring. My daughter's godmother furnished her first home with thrift store finds lovingly refinished. In the past, things were built to last. It is this sense of solidity which the old imparts to the new.

HANDCRAFTS

Crafts

～

BY KATE STRASBURG

Another source of comfort in design comes from craft. Our Healing Environments showcase is filled with handmade things, as is The Healing Home. I recently purchased a miniature basket, painstakingly woven by hand in an Asian country. What does this tiny object do for me? It speaks of patience and integrity. It was made in a context of tradition, rather than with an eye for profit. It has been made this way for centuries. It is reminiscent of an earlier age when time was not at a premium. When the rhythms of life were tied to the earth. When man was not the measure of all things. It speaks to me and tells me that all my hurrying cannot affect the universe. It tells me to take a deep breath and slow down.

OUR NEW HOME

A New Incarnation

BY KATE STRASBURG

Although the average American moves five times in a lifetime, many of us cling as fondly to the status quo as our European counterparts. There is nothing in the Western tradition which instructs, as Buddhism does, that change is constant and, therefore, excessive attachment a certain cause of unhappiness. However if we view crises from an Asian perspective, they each provide a unique opportunity for transformation. As the ancient Chinese *I Ching* proclaims: chaos paves the way for creation.

The process of reconfiguring a dream does not come easily. I am reminded of something I read about transformation in O *Magazine*. When a caterpillar creates a chrysalis, it does not simply affix wings to its body. It must first lose all semblance of caterpillar before reemerging as butterfly. The process of transformation takes a great deal of faith. One must let go of all that has been before reinventing oneself. As André Gide wrote: "One does not discover new lands without consenting to lose all sight of shore at first and for a long time."

And so when Traci and I realized that Healing Environments would have to find a new home, as rents were rising and the troubled economy depleting non-profits' funding, we entered a passage of unknowing. For nine years our nonprofit's identity had been fused with our twelve-room showcase in Palo Alto. How could it possibly be preserved in a much smaller space in San Francisco? The journey was not an easy one, but what we emerged with is far more magical than that which we left behind. The caterpillar has indeed become a butterfly.

Our new space on Sacramento Street in San Francisco is a fraction of the space we had previously. Yet the impact we have has expanded geometrically. Located in a former antique store in one of San Francisco's loveliest neighborhoods, we find ourselves encircled by healthcare facilities.

When Traci arrived she began leaving journals out in front of our storefront in a wooden rack. They disappeared at a heartening rate. We even began to feel that our presence in a commercial area offered a spiritual antidote to those seeking relief in excessive consumption.

One gentleman brought a friend to simply experience the space. "I'm hoping if he can just be present, he will realize what is missing from his life," he said.

Let me describe the space in more detail and the process of transforming it.

When Traci takes on a design job she steadfastly refuses to do design boards. The reason being that we believe in the creative process as an organic one. I am reminded of Christopher Alexander, the eccentric and innovative architect who allows the land to "speak" to him when designing a building. So Traci and I moved into Sacramento Street with only a rough idea of what would go where and how it would all work out.

Let me share with you an example of how leaving space for inspiration can result in magic. The centerpiece of our Palo Alto space had been a magnificent antique hand-carved African door. A symbol of transformation, it never failed to inspire our visitors. Traci and I had placed most of our furniture in the new front room when we realized we had failed to find a spot for our most prized possession. I wandered into one of the two back rooms. A small alcove in one would have to replace our meditation room in Palo Alto. We had placed a small Asian trunk in it, with a beautiful Mexican reproduction of an antique cross and a lovely cast of a cherub's head and wings. Clearly the door completed the vignette. Just after we had placed it there, one of the movers entered the room. Unaware of our mission and engaged in a far from spiritual profession, he provided all the validation we needed for our choice. Glancing at the trio of transcendent objects he gasped audibly.

Later we would add the manzanita branches from our first fundraiser, still graced with the Tibetan prayer bells, hand calligraphed poems and diaphanous ribbons left there in memory of loved ones. The resulting meditation alcove is far more powerful than our previous one.

Similarly, a small open closet became a second memorial space, a place for visitors to light candles in memory of loved ones. Once again, serendipity played a major role in its creation. Two other of our favorite objects were difficult to place. They are both extremely colorful, yet we prefer an earthy, more neutral palette. Both hold special meaning for us. One is a traditional Mexican tree of life, created by a patient with no prior art experience. The other a small yet vibrant lap quilt sewn by my cousin Eleanor, a quilt designer, for a dear friend she lost to AIDS.

The final piece of the memorial alcove came together when a mover placed a small round table with a copper top in the closet to get it out of the way. The perfect fireproof surface for votive candles. A nondescript closet became a colorful, meaning-filled memorial.

A third installment of design by inspiration occurred after Traci and I did a table for Dining by Design, the AIDS fundraiser cosponsored by Elle Decor and Taittinger Champagne. Wanting to create a table that would authentically portray our mission, we chose the theme "Dark Night of the Soul." On a black silk tablecloth we placed an exquisite ancient gilded wooden Kuan Yin (the Buddhist Bodhisattva of compassion) flanked with large black vases filled with flame-red spider orchids.

Wanting to represent our ecumenical stance accurately as well, we placed an Ethiopian Coptic cross and a beautiful menorah by the sculptor Erté on the other side of the table. After the event we brought all three religious icons back to the office, not sure of where they would find a home. In a matter of minutes they transformed the front room into a powerfully spiritual presence on Sacramento Street.

Moving as Transformation

ॐ

BY TRACI TERAOKA

In 2003, Kate and I had decided to let go of our original Healing Environments location of nine years—our founding nest for the mission of our work. Believe me, it wasn't easy coming to that decision. It can be very difficult to imagine life differently. I am certain that we had to go through many stages of grieving to let go, finally.

So, the search began. We optimistically saw space after space—and we were often confronted with different issues of why each space would or wouldn't work. The process reminded me of what we experienced the first time around in 1993, with each physical space shaping the opportunity—and with us always staying true to what is essential to our mission, reviewing what could be flexible and what was non-negotiable. We had hoped that by making the decision to let go and embrace the future—the right solution would appear alongside our intention. We must have looked at well over 40 places over several months; all the while trying fresh perspectives, envisioning our intention to help the suffering with beauty and comfort.

Kate and I were getting edgy, as well as supremely frustrated and tired. I asked her if we could switch gears and try something different—collage. I wanted to pause and play, even if it didn't yield anything. Within two days, we had a large black box that, when opened, revealed wishes and hopes for the new space. I put my own collages in the box and kept it near as we began a new pursuit now with the deadline for moving out of our original space fast approaching.

How frustrating to try to let go—reaching for the new shore—having a vision of what it might look like and then realizing "wrong shore." Our faith and hope had to become yet more consciously activated and practiced.

Of course now that we can look back on the situation, we can see the grace and eventual good fortune we found. I think Kate and I found comfort in our both being flexible about how the mission and work could continue in many different forms. We "tried on" several reincarnations and in the end—it really seems that despite the hardships and stress, hope and faith were rejuvenated time and again—when we moved in early August, there was a natural fit where we landed. In fact, many folks have walked into the new space experiencing it as a refuge—feeling as if it had been there for ages. And it really does feel like that.

For those of you experiencing the challenges of change we send you hope—realize where you yourself are "stuck" in a mindset that isn't helping you move on. There is a terrific Buddhist visualization for letting go of feelings and experiences that we are clinging to, which I would like to share with you here. Imagine yourself walking through a room full of balloons. As you walk through the room imagine letting yourself reach for different balloons, holding and letting go of each one until you are on the other side of the room. Each balloon represents one of the many experiences that make up who we are and become our individual life experience. Are you intentionally holding one balloon, holding on to it for dear life, passing many other experiences and feelings that are available if only you could loosen your grip? The idea is to let yourself have many experiences and to practice reaching for and letting go of these opportunities to experience fully what is intended for you in your own unique life.

If Kate and I had held on to only one possibility—if we hadn't created both mental and heart space for change—we would not be in this new blessed space with access to so many healthcare facilities. Now we have an office that presents a whole new range of possibilities to help people. The space is smaller—but that's ok—the work itself is immense and unlimited by the walls that surround it. We are able to demonstrate how our environment affects us—to inspire, to meet emotional and spiritual needs with beauty, art, comfort and meaning. It is a lending library—encompassing such topics as health and nutrition, spirituality and religion, art and design, creativity, and living and dying, as well as a space for ritual and remembrance. Ordinary people walk up to the storefront expecting an antique store, and are usually pleasantly surprised when they realize we don't sell anything. In fact, with 28 journals created in the last nine years—we are often handing things out free of any charge or expectation.

It has been heartening to have someone walk up—curious about what they see—inquire if they can browse—realize they cannot shop, instead connect—and to have their reply be, "Perfect," or, "This is what I really needed." Or, "I just helped my mom die—could I spend some time here? I feel like I have been walking around in an altered state that no one could possibly understand."

I have moved twice in the last three years. And, as I write this piece, I have learned I will need to make an additional move before I can be "settled." I am the type of person who generally likes change. I enjoy the process of seeing the possibility in all things and the way old things can come together with a fresh perspective, but not quite at this rate. It can feel out of control and scary—yet, I trust that relatively soon I will be able to look back on this chapter of my life as being difficult and that I was able to survive it with grace.

TOUR

A Tour of the Original Healing Environments

BY KATE STRASBURG

Before moving to San Francisco in 2003 Healing Environments was located in Palo Alto, California for nine years. This farewell tour was tape-recorded as a means of preserving the original space.

Welcome to Healing Environments. We always start our tour by giving a little bit of background about how we came to create Healing Environments. I had lost a great number of loved ones to cancer—both of my parents died of cancer and, in my late forties, I lost three very close friends in just 18 months. I desperately wanted to do something with my loss to turn it into something positive, into a gift back to the world.

Then Traci and I met. We connected over our tremendous love of design and were united in our desire to use this love of design for a higher purpose. Partly because of her age and her contacts, whereas I was moved by people struggling with cancer, Traci connected with people who were struggling with AIDS. And so we came upon the mission of Healing Environments which is to relieve

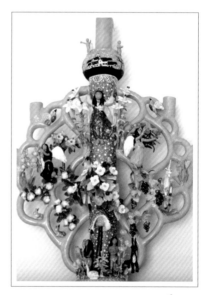

figure 1

the suffering of those seriously ill, not only with cancer and AIDS but with all kinds of illness.

In this first room of Healing Environments, we're in a mock art studio. We believe very firmly in the power of art to transform suffering—not only viewing art, but creating art. We have some outstanding examples in this art room. I'm looking now at an incredible Tree of Life which was made out of pâpier-maché by an Hispanic gentleman whom we met in a store of Mexican art (fig. 1). When we complimented him on this and said we'd like to purchase it, he said that it was his own creation. He had spent six months in the hospital and with absolutely no prior art experience, had taught himself the art of pâpier-maché and created this wonderful work of art. He told us that he would like to teach other patients how to work with pâpier-maché as well.

Traci and I have a theory that there is an artist in each one of us if we can silence the inner critic, which appears in our culture at about age six when children start saying, "Oh, that doesn't look like a real this or that," or "I can't draw." This beautiful example of folk art is a stunning example of everyone's artistic capability.

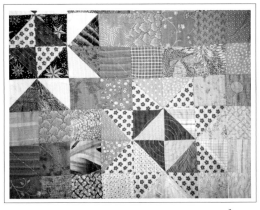

figure 2

The other moving exhibit that we have in this room is a lap quilt (fig. 2), which my cousin, who was an off-Broadway costume designer, created for her best friend who was dying of AIDS. She made it small so he could cover his lap in a wheelchair. When he died, she created a baby quilt out of his favorite shirts in his memory and gave it to a baby with AIDS. So that was what she did with her grief over the loss of her dear friend.

Another exhibit in this first room is a small chest which we have hanging on the wall (fig. 3). One of our great concerns about hospitalization is how impersonal it is. Doctor Thomas Delbanco of Beth Israel Deaconess Medical Center in Boston says this depersonalization has serious psychological impact which affects physical outcomes. We believe that patients suffer greatly because the first thing that happens to you when you enter a hospital is that they take away everything that tells you who you are—they take your clothes, your jewelry, any objects that have any value or

meaning whatsoever. So we would love to see some kind of system by which hospitals could have on display items and artifacts that have great significance to a patient. One of our favorite hospitals in Hawaii, North Hawaii Community Hospital, has beautiful niches in the rooms which can be used for art and flowers, religious icons and personal

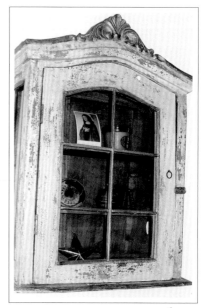

figure 3

items. We believe every patient should have some symbolic representation of who he is and what is important to him.

Another item of significance in this room is a comfort quilt. One of our cancer patients had been given a very bad prognosis. She had just moved here with her husband from Michigan. She had only been here three weeks when she was told that she had colon cancer and a very poor chance of surviving. Her entire support system, meanwhile, was back in Michigan 2000 miles away. So what we suggested to her was that she take this quilt—I wish you could feel it—it's very soft and lightweight, made in India. We had Eleanor, my cousin, make two dozen bluebirds out of this fabric which is self-adhesive—you merely iron it on (fig. 4). Our cancer patient sent these bluebirds to two dozen of her friends and family in Michigan with instructions that they should write messages of love and encouragement on the bluebirds,

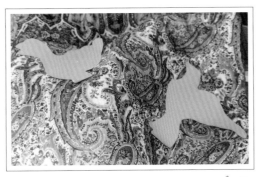

figure 4

which were then ironed on to the quilt. And in the great tradition of quilts, which were often made by women to encourage each other in difficult times, she had the comfort of friends and family symbolically supporting her in the West.

Another object we have in this small art studio is an art cart. Now this is not a unique idea—art carts do exist in hospitals, but we have had quite a few hospital administrators comment that ours is particularly patient-friendly. I think this is because it's made out of natural wood and has baskets on it instead of being made out of metal. It has an assortment of videos, CDs, reading materials, and personal journals—healing tools to pass out to patients and caregivers. So those are the high points of the art studio.

You'll notice in Healing Environments that in terms of signage, we decided to give each room a name that is a verb, and the name of the art studio is *Create*. I'd also like to read the plaques to you. We have two marble plaques. One reads:

Healing Environments
A sanctuary for those who are suffering,
a shrine for those who have suffered,
a showcase for ways to relieve suffering,
for we are not alone.

The other plaque reads:

To those who have died alone,
to those who have died well loved,
to those who have died in pain,
to those who have died in peace,
to those who have died with lives fulfilled,
to those who have died with dreams unlived,
Healing Environments is dedicated
to the relief of all suffering
for we are one.

Even in the bathroom we have healing art. We have a framed print of a painting by Keith Smith whom I met at Commonweal. Keith lost his wife to cancer. He loved her dearly and he spent the two years following her death painting his grief and writing poetry about his loss. This print (fig. 5) shows an empty bed with one pillow that's been slept on recently and the other not, and healing plants growing up over the bed. Keith actually published his poetry and his art in a book called *Mourning Sickness*. As much as he adored his wife, by immersing himself in his grief so productively and creatively for two years, he was able to fall in love again and happily remarry, although he had thought he would never love again.

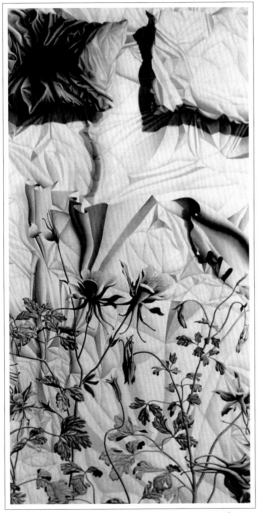

figure 5

Now we're moving into the main hall and we have this magnificent African door which is one of our very favorite artifacts in Healing Environments (fig. 6). We love the symbolism of the door because it can be read at so many different levels. If one believes in life after death, the door can be seen as a transition to another life. If one doesn't believe in life after death, it can be read simply as transition or transformation. We placed a wonderful hand-carved Indian door at the beginning of the corridor at the Wing's Cancer Clinic in Memphis, Tennessee. It is a strong symbol for cancer patients embarking on their transformative journey.

Now the main room in Healing Environments is an art gallery, and the word that we have here on the wall is *Contemplate*. You'll see a number of manzanita branches which are hung with beautiful diaphanous ribbons and Tibetan prayer bells which

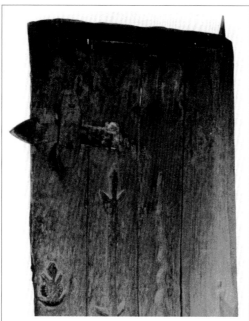

figure 6

I love the African door because its symbolic carved figures of animals—a snake, a lizard, a turtle—link nature with the sacred rituals of everyday. It has a wonderful arrow-like latch that feels good to the hand. So that's another aspect of what should be added into healthcare environments and into our own homes. Items that are real and meaningful.

Traci Teraoka

have poetry hanging from their clappers. At our first fundraiser, we put these manzanita branches in the far corner of my garden in a private area, and invited people during the night to remember loved ones they had lost either with bells or with ribbons. Although Traci and I were not conscious of anyone actively doing that, at the end of the evening, we went back and found every bell and every ribbon had been used in this way. We have not wanted to dismantle them (fig. 7). They are precious and holy to us and beautiful symbols of how ritual can be healing. The Wing's Cancer Clinic did a similar project with their cancer patients for the new year. They had them attach prayers to a large archway. As I've said, we're great believers in ritual.

The art in this room is also symbolic. We believe that healing art is art which addresses the depth of the patient experience. Decorative art is nice, but we don't think that it can

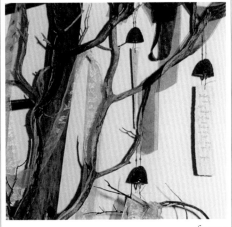

figure 7

Giving people something to connect to, something that brings them some peace, something that brings them a sense of the world being larger outside of their crisis. That's really important.

Traci Teraoka

speak to a patient in terms of what that patient is going through. These photographs were all taken on a Swedish island. One is of a stairway ascending out in nature. The center one is of a tree, looking up into its branches. When I was at Commonweal, they suggested that if we wanted to help patients, we needed to think of ourselves as trees drawing energy from the universe, not giving our own personal energy, but drawing energy from the universe which then we could transmit to patients. If one gives one's own personal energy, then one will eventually burn out. The third photograph is of a path wending its way around through trees, around a large cliff, and you can't see where the path is leading, which to us is symbolic of life's journey. These are all examples of what we consider to be healing art. We also have other symbols in the room—a ladder and another photograph of a small window which is evocative again, looking out on nothing in particular, just letting the light in. We also have a large, decorative mirror, which is symbolic of reflection or identity.

The next room that I'm going to talk about is a double bedroom which we call *Rest*. When we set up Healing Environments, we wanted to create fictional patients' rooms. We believe healing environments, ideally, would be as individualized as the patients themselves. We created this beautiful white bedroom (fig. 8), which is everyone's favorite, in memory of a young woman who died of AIDS at age 26. She was a very wealthy New Yorker and was one of the first women to have AIDS when everyone thought it was a gay man's disease. She went to all the high schools in New York and said, "Well, if I can have AIDS, then you are all in danger, too." Unfortunately, the poor young woman contracted it in her first sexual encounter with a bisexual bartender at the age of 16 and she died at 26. But in this bedroom, we have made her very spiritual—not religious but spiritual. She draws on our fictionalized version of her life as someone brought up Catholic who rediscovers and renews the faith of her youth in a very personal way. The light in this room is particularly out-

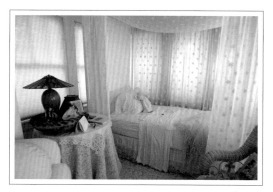

figure 8

standing. It comes in the late afternoon through these beautiful diaphanous curtains and it's quite otherworldly. Now, not everyone would want an all-white bedroom if they were dying. We happen to think it's quite heavenly. The ideal healing environment would be one which suits the individual perfectly. The young woman's Jungian sandtray, which is on her bedside table, symbolizes the horror of her disease: the doll house bride is being carried off by the monster lizard (fig. 9). He is carrying off her hopes and dreams for she will in fact never marry.

In the center of the sand-tray we have her as a small child with her mother, a beautiful dancing dress from her teenage years, and then the portend of what's to come: a skull of an animal, a tombstone. And then, because she does have faith in life after death, there's a small church and a Mexican foil cathedral which symbolizes eternity.

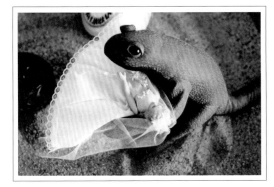

figure 9

One of the wonderful ideas which we've gleaned from real life is a prayer schedule. The son of my ex-husband's best friend was paralyzed from the neck down in a touch football game at Stanford. His friends signed up for an hour of the day, and they promised that at that hour, be it 1:00 p.m. or 1:00 a.m., they would send him love or, if they were religious, pray for him. He had this prayer schedule by his bed and he could wake up anytime and know that this friend or that friend was thinking of him or praying for him. We thought this was a beautiful concrete expression of support.

Next to the bed, on the chair, we have the knitting that I actually did while my father was dying. I found the most beautiful, soft mohair yarn that I could and started a sweater for each of my children. I would sit by my father's bedside, and knit, and pray as I knit each stitch. I found it incredibly calming. We also have in this room a very soothing Japanese-style painting of two deer.

We have quite an extensive collection of videos and audiotapes. They are for entertainment as well as inspiration, for education as well as visualization. A lot of them are spiritual. We try to meet all belief systems as well as have inspirational offerings for people who are not spiritual. There's a surprising amount of inspirational material available. One of our favorite videos is of the group of women that sang choral music to keep their morale up in Japanese prisoner of war camps in the Philippines.

We also have a favorite Thomas Wolfe quote which I had copied in calligraphy for a dear friend of mine who was dying. It begins: *Something has spoken to me in the night…* and appears on the cover of one of our journals. It's very inspiring.

On the chaise lounge (fig. 10) which is quite lovely, we have the mohair throw that I gave my dying mother-in-law who was like a mother to me. The other bed in this area is for a fictional middle-aged, workaholic male who neglected his family in his ambition

and now that he's dying, finds that they are not there for him. When we were bringing a widow through Healing Environments she started to cry because this patient reminded her of her deceased husband, who had worked too hard at the expense of his family. Unfortunately, this patient is much more typical than our young woman who has great spiritual resources.

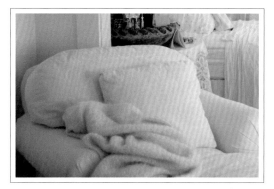

figure 10

Moving on to the next room which is entitled *Store*, this is our storeroom (fig. 11). One of our very first consulting jobs was with the Cancer Center at Marin General Hospital. They wanted to set up a resource center and we showed them this room. This is what we wish hospital gift shops looked like. It has a large selection of books, a variety of blank journals and very meaningful greeting cards. We think it's quite difficult to find a card for someone who does not have a chance of getting well, so we collected the ones we thought were wonderful. And we have a number of healing tools: magnificent Mexican cathedral candles, Indian massage oil, meaningful dog tags which are also on display in the other room. They're copper and have words on them such as *faith*, *hope* and *love*. One cancer patient saw them and said, "What I need is a miracle." We brought her into the storeroom and, sure enough, there was a dog tag with the word *miracle* on it. Now we don't want you to think we encourage magical thinking, but we do believe that sometimes the spirit can rally and the

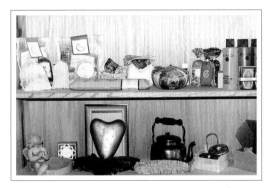

figure 11

immune system can be mobilized with blessed results. However this subject is sensitive because the patients who aren't able to go into remission should never feel that they failed in any way. It's just a blessing when it happens.

Another example of our belief in intention is that we have ritual kits. We had the idea that if patients had individualized ritual kits, they could take them to the hospital with them and that ritual could help ground them. When I went to Greece, I didn't want to be away from Healing Environments. At that time we had a young man who was working for us, David, and he and I used to meditate every morning at 9 o'clock. We figured out that 9:00 a.m. in California was 6:00 p.m. in Greece, and so I took a ritual kit with me and we both meditated at the same time everyday even though we were half a world apart. So we at Healing Environments like rituals that overcome time and space. The ritual kit that I created for sustaining myself through the pain of divorce could also be modified for someone struggling with illness or someone supporting someone dealing with illness. We encourage people to be creative in this way. So that's the storeroom.

Now we're moving into the next room, which is entitled *Play* and *Meditate*. This building is beautifully suited to our needs because each room has alcoves, and we've placed our meditation room in one of these alcoves. We have Japanese tatami mats on

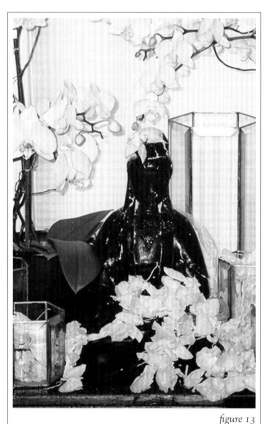

figure 13

I often suggest adding a sculpture, a fountain, or other elements of nature. Such a room can offer solace, a place to pray, a place to feel safe. It can be a place of inspiration.

TRACI TERAOKA

the floor, we have a fountain. When we had Japanese visitors, they told us that in Japan the sound of running water is considered very healing and we agree. We have a Kuan Yin (fig. 13) which is a Buddhist symbol of compassion. In our meditation room, we tried to be ecumenical, but it's difficult to represent all religions, so we picked the Kuan Yin because she is so tranquil. We wish hospitals were more dedicated to creating a space that feels sacred. We believe this space does with white orchids arching overhead, the sound of running water, beautiful green plants, and bare branches in an ancient vase. We have two large candles on stands. Our intention was to light one daily for cancer patients, one daily for AIDS patients.

The front part of the room entitled *Play* is our sandtray room. Jungian sandtray technique is used by therapists to access the subconscious directly. We have several thousand objects that Traci and I have col-lected. Sandtray objects are objects which have a high emotional valence, that is, which are highly evocative. Our absolute favorite object is also our least expensive and our most powerful—that's this broken doll which had its legs broken off before we bought it. We got it for $2. Her chest looks as though it's been painted with gentian violet in preparation for surgery. This is an extremely powerful and very inexpensive object. Our objects come from doll house stores and many other sources. Again, most of them are very evocative. I'm looking at an eight ball, a Mexican skull, a little teddy bear that has broken its leg, war medals including the purple heart, a very battered and torn *E.T.*

A friend of my daughter's came and did a sandtray, and she picked out the following items: she chose a gun and said this is for the violence in my life; she picked out an egg timer and said this is for time running out;

she picked out a compass and said this is for my lack of direction; she represented herself as a very winsome fairy in the center of the sandtray, and then she picked out a house and said, "This is my home but it's broken. I wish that there was a way of showing that it's broken." So we got a cookie jar that's a house and the roof comes off. Actually the process isn't supposed to be as conscious as she made it. You're supposed to pick the objects you're drawn to and not analyze why, then place them in the sand without conscious thought. When you step back and reflect, what you have in front of you is a map of your subconscious issues.

The sandtray that we have on display was done by my daughter (fig. 15). There are three eggs and a little turtle is hatching out of one. My daughter was pregnant at the time but did not know it consciously. That shows you something of the power of this technique! At Commonweal in Bolinas,

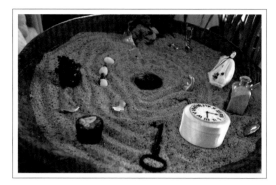

figure 15

California, they have the patients who come for week-long retreats make a sandtray at the beginning of their stay. Then a week later they make a second one and they often see that they've made a great deal of spiritual progress. One woman in particular, at the beginning of her stay, saw her illness as the enemy, and had little toy soldiers and guns trying to fight it. At the end of her week, she saw it as a jewel that was bringing her a gift of self-awareness and personal growth.

One more thing in this room that is wonderful is this piece of art which I purchased after my divorce (fig. 16). I was a German major in college and it's a German love letter. The reason I love it is because you can barely read it. My son had dyslexia and poor handwriting as many dyslexic children do because of their difficulty with hand-eye coordination. When he saw it, he said, "Mom, why did you frame that scribble scrabble?" and I said, "Well, Greg, a teacher might call it that, but actually this is a work art. You're right, it is writing and I consider it very beautiful!" When I told that story to the gallery owner, he gave me a big hug because he, too, was dyslexic and he, too, had been criticized severely by his teacher for his handwriting. That's a very good example of the healing power of art.

So, moving on, now we're going in the back of the building. There's a very strong monotype by an artist friend of mine who later committed suicide. It's of an impressionistic cross with barbed wire symbolically around the bottom of the cross and wings at the juncture of the crosspiece.

Moving into the dining room, which we named *Nourish*, we have three large black and white nature photographs here. They're from a book called *Here Today*, which was taken from *Here today, gone tomorrow*. They are all pictures of endangered species, and we'd been doing these tours for four years before one of the patients said, "Endangered species, that's what *we* are." And we realized that symbolism works on amazing levels. Sometimes you're not at all conscious of it.

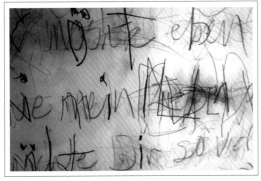

figure 16

There's a tender close-up of a kit fox, just the face of the tranquilized fox looking very benign, a beautiful photograph of an oak tree, and another one of a pelican. We also have an Indonesian weaving called an *ikat* which is symbolic of creation (fig. 17).

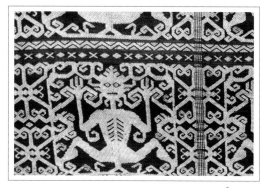

figure 17

And, again, we believe very strongly in ritual. When our publication mailing list grew to 10,000, we had a little ceremony. We had one large candle and four small ones for the four of us who work on it. The silver holders are engraved *10,000 lights* to symbolize our 10,000 readers.

We love antiques. You'll notice that throughout Healing Environments we have many antiques and also a lot of ethnic art. We love ethnic art because we believe that it is so strong symbolically that it's grounding. And antiques are grounding because they, too, are a symbol of survival, of the transcendence of time.

Moving into the library, the word on the library wall is, of course, *Read*. Around the library (fig. 18), we have some prints which we got from a reproduction of a beautiful medieval book. A very large book, it was $80 in a used book shop. We framed many of the pages. We love them because they are medieval, they're in Latin, and so they are quite mysterious to anybody who does not read Latin, and the only hint of what their content is that one of the pages is entitled *Chartres*. They are in fact descriptions of cities that existed in the Middle Ages. They are classically framed and a good example of how art can be inexpensive and quite wonderful.

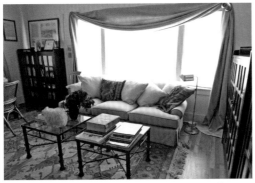

So we want to create peaceful, meaningful environments with offerings—ethnic, cultural and artistic— that make us feel more connected to our world. Anxiety in a room can be contagious. Places that are comfortable to sit in, comfortable to be in and feel welcoming, these are things that would make a huge difference in our healthcare environments.

TRACI TERAOKA

We have quite a resource library. We have books on Western and Eastern medicine, books on spirituality, and because we believe that the healing process should not be isolated from life, we also have books on relationship, poetry, art and architecture.

There's a very wonderful story about the library. I have what I call a book angel. I've written about it for *A Light in the Mist*. It's a little far out, but I have to tell you this one story. We desperately needed a quote about Buddhism once and we had no idea where to find it. We needed the Buddhist definition of *maitri* which in Sanskrit means *compassionate friendship*. I stood in front of these bookshelves and I asked the universe to help me find it. I opened the spirituality bookshelf and without hesitation went to a book I'd never read, and again without pausing opened it to page 148. And there was exactly what we needed: the Buddha's explanation of *maitri* or *compassionate friendship*.

So moving on to the kitchen, the sign in the kitchen is *Compose*. The Planetree model and others have recognized the role of the kitchen in nourishing body and soul. We designed this kitchen on a low budget, and it's quite reassuring to see what a good eye can do with not very much money.

Moving to our last room, our office, which is of course named *Work*. We have perhaps the most beautiful piece of art in the entire center here—this sculpture of one man compassionately consoling another (fig. 19). It's so beautiful that Maitri had an artist draw it for their logo. When Traci was giving her father a tour, when he saw this statue, he put his hand on the bronze and said, "This is what it's all about." That is a perfect example of how the right piece of art can speak volumes and can say more about mission than very long mission statements and business plans.

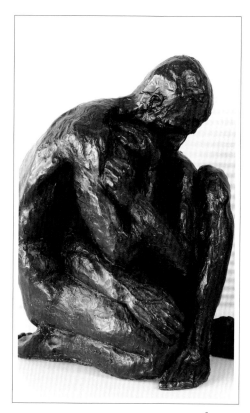

figure 19

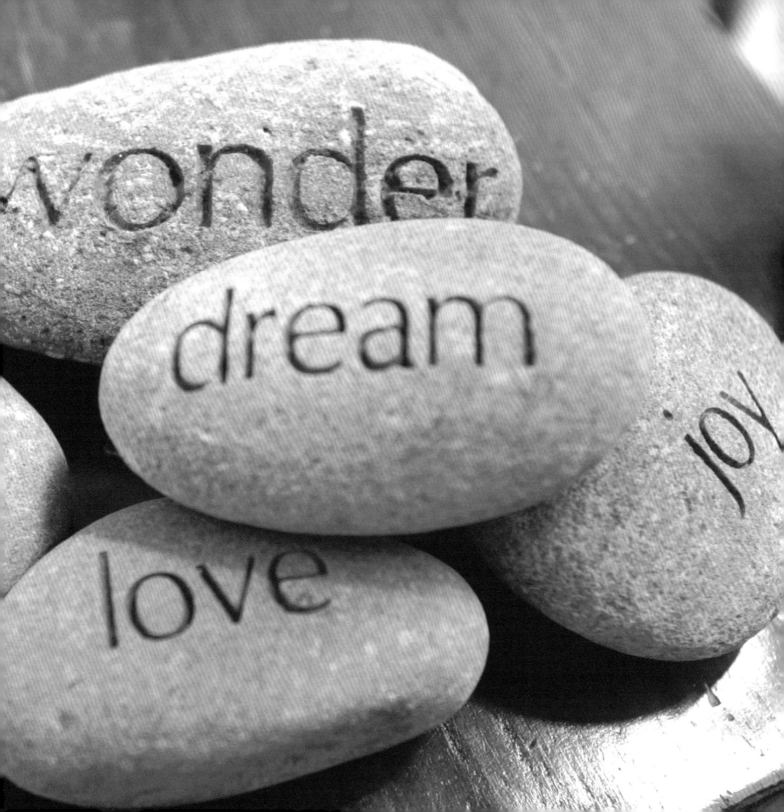

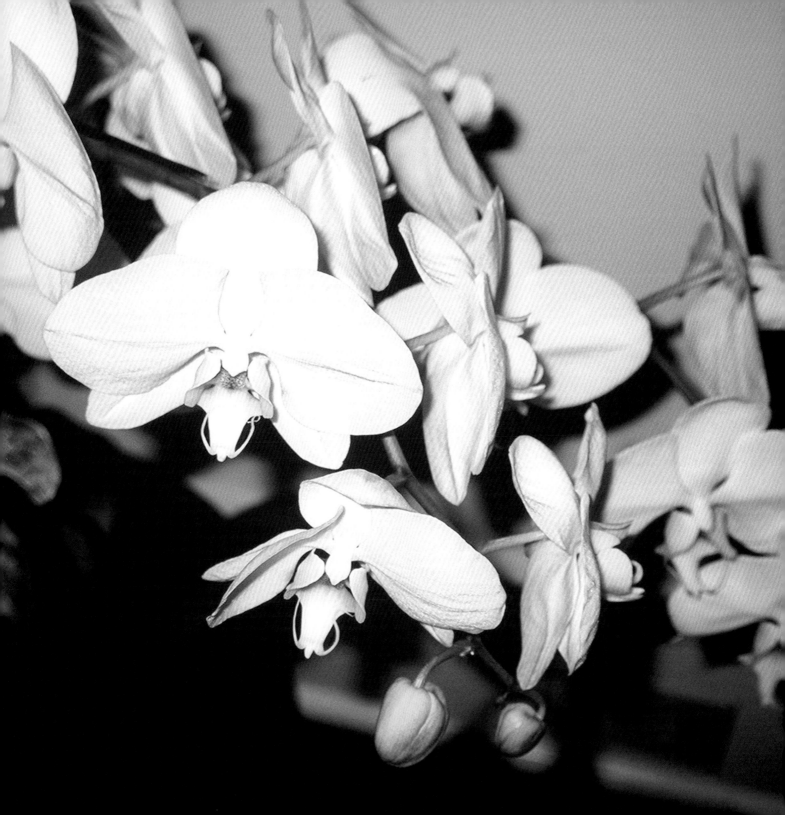

PORTFOLIO

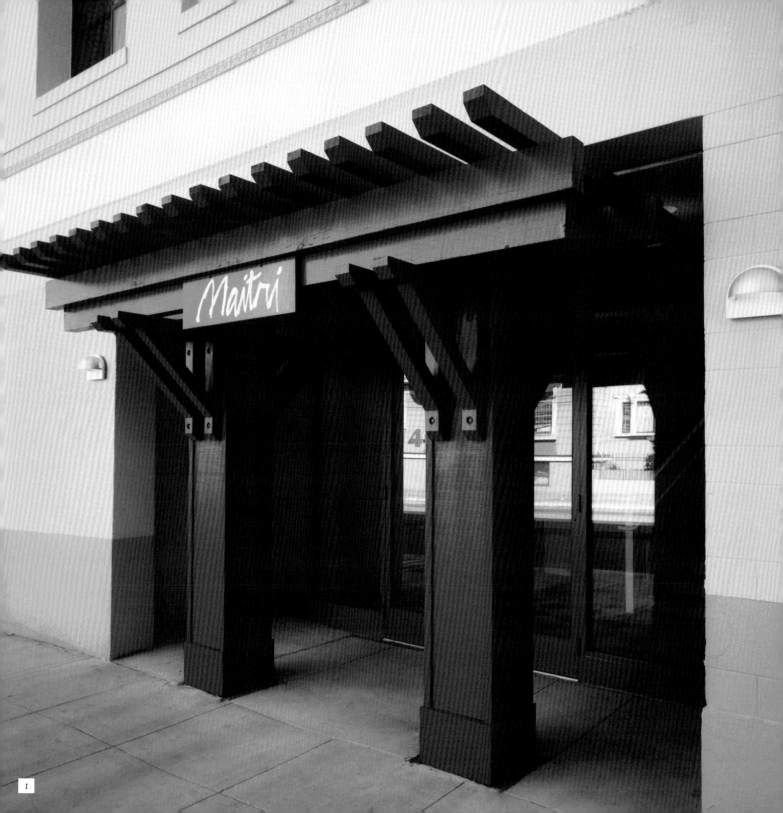

MAITRI

RESIDENTIAL AIDS FACILITY

SAN FRANCISCO, CALIFORNIA

Maitri Residential AIDS Facility
San Francisco, California

Formerly a Zen hospice housed in a San Francisco Victorian, today Maitri is a fifteen bedroom residential care facility for people living with AIDS. Deriving its name from the Buddhist concept of compassionate care, Maitri extends the comfort of a homelike as well as spiritual setting to its residents. In order to honor the philosophy of Maitri, designer Traci Teraoka chose a collection of Asian art and antiques for the common rooms. Each bedroom is a unique offering of warm wood furnishings. The residents take pride as well as comfort in the beauty and expression of their surroundings.

IMAGE INDEX:

1. Entrance   2. Stair Mural   3. Public Living Room   4. Resident Room
5. Resident Room   6. Meditation Room

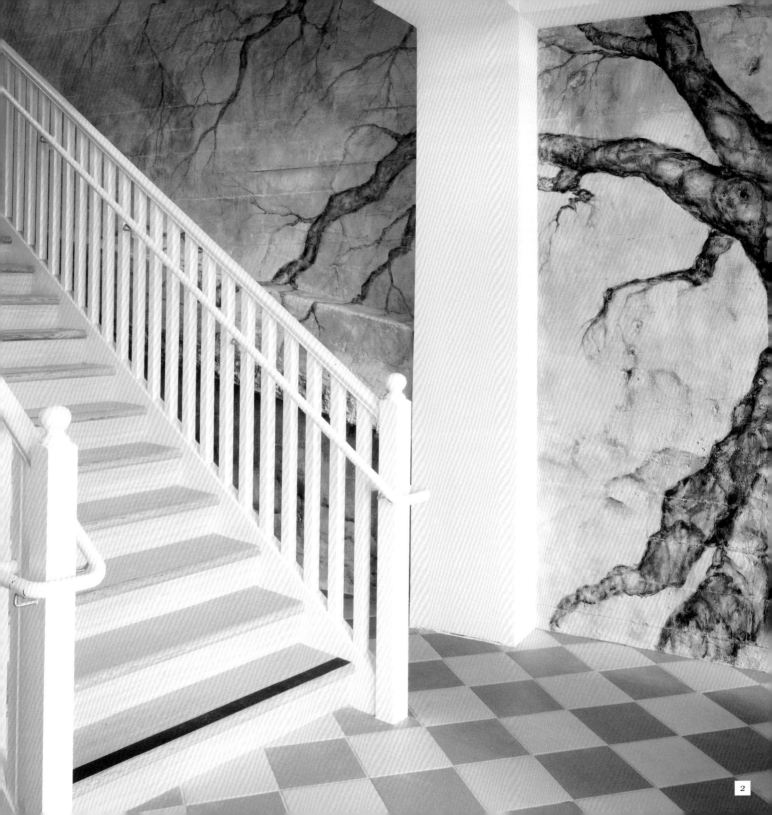

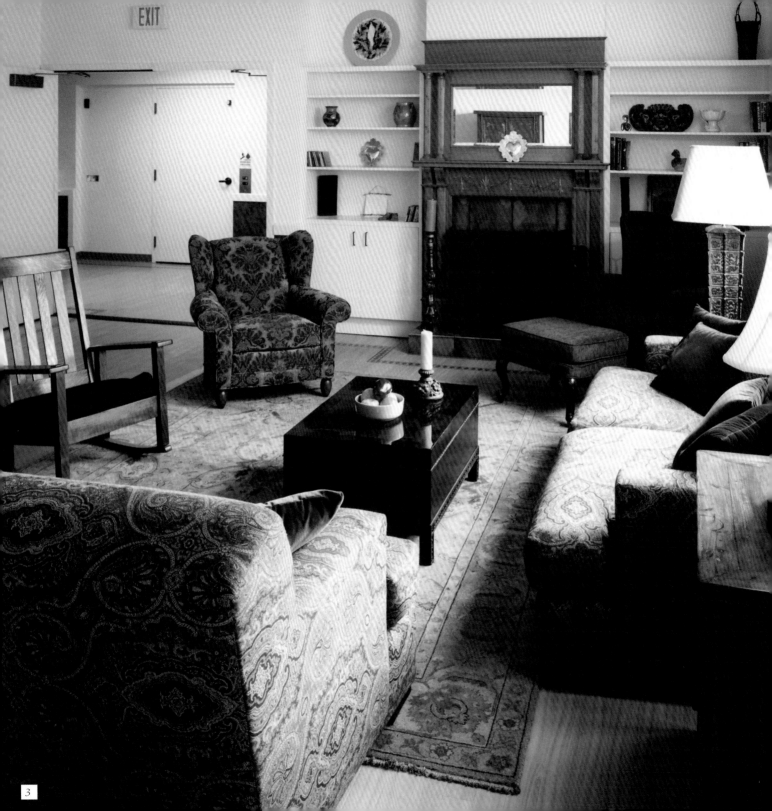

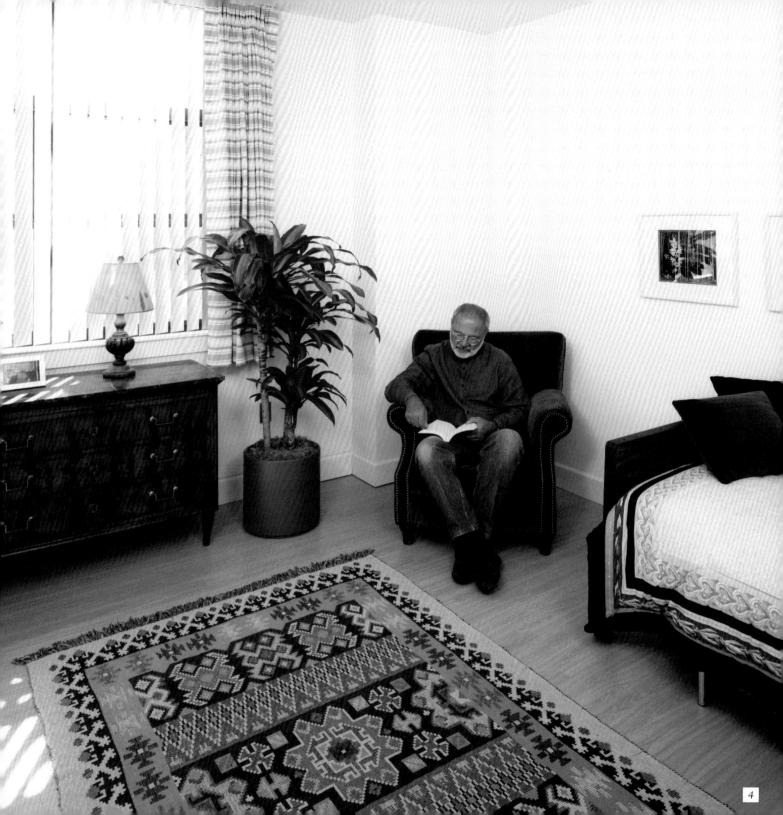

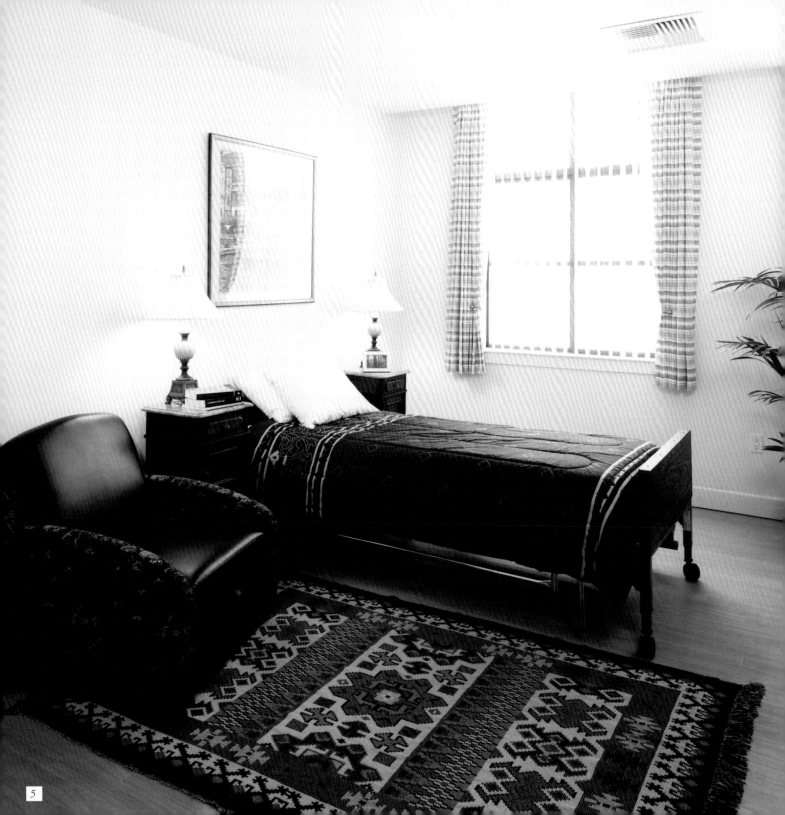

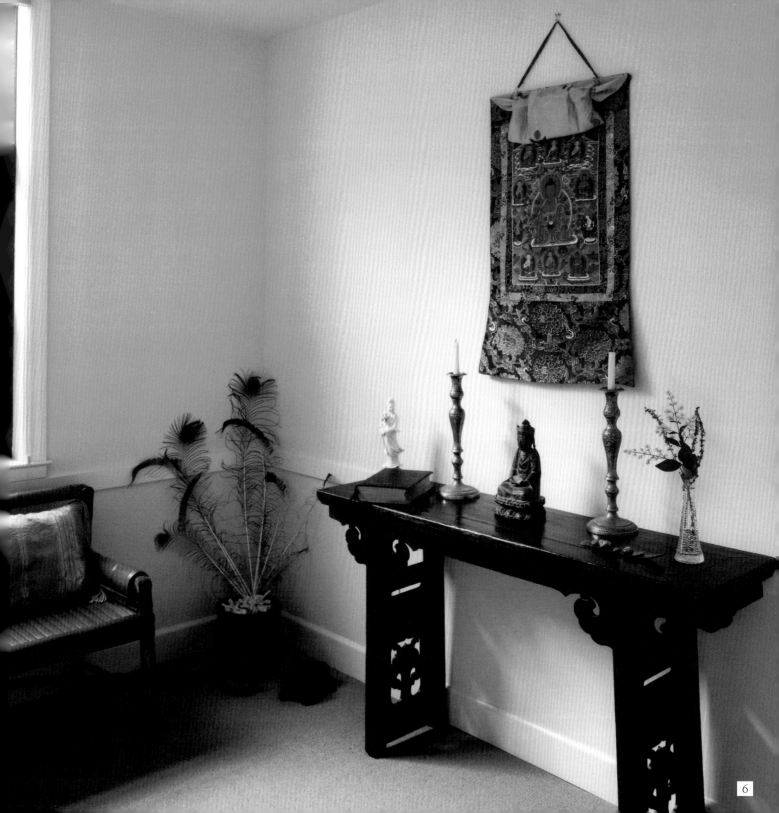

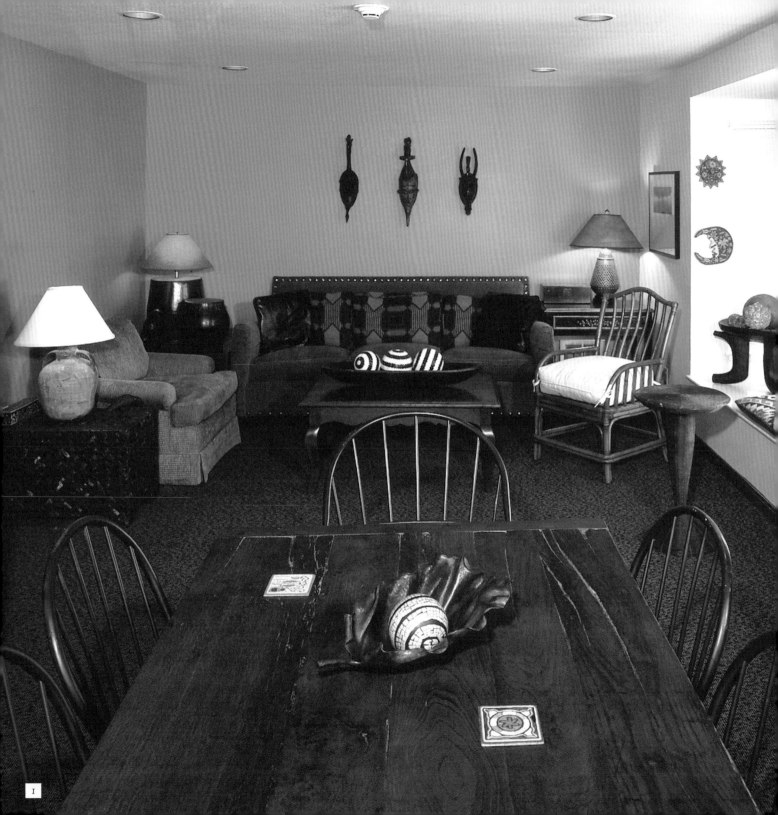

BRANDY MOORE-RAFIKI HOUSE
RESIDENTIAL AIDS FACILITY
SAN FRANCISCO, CALIFORNIA

Brandy Moore-Rafiki House
Residential AIDS Facility
San Francisco, California

A project of the Black Coalition on AIDS, Rafiki House is another pro bono design installation created by Healing Environments. Heeding the staff's desire that it reflect the African heritage of its residents, Traci filled Rafiki with strong color and vibrant folk art. The result is a strong, life-affirming statement for this eleven bedroom residential care facility for people living with AIDS.

IMAGE INDEX:

1. Living Room   2. Therapy Room   3. Therapy Room   4. Dining Room

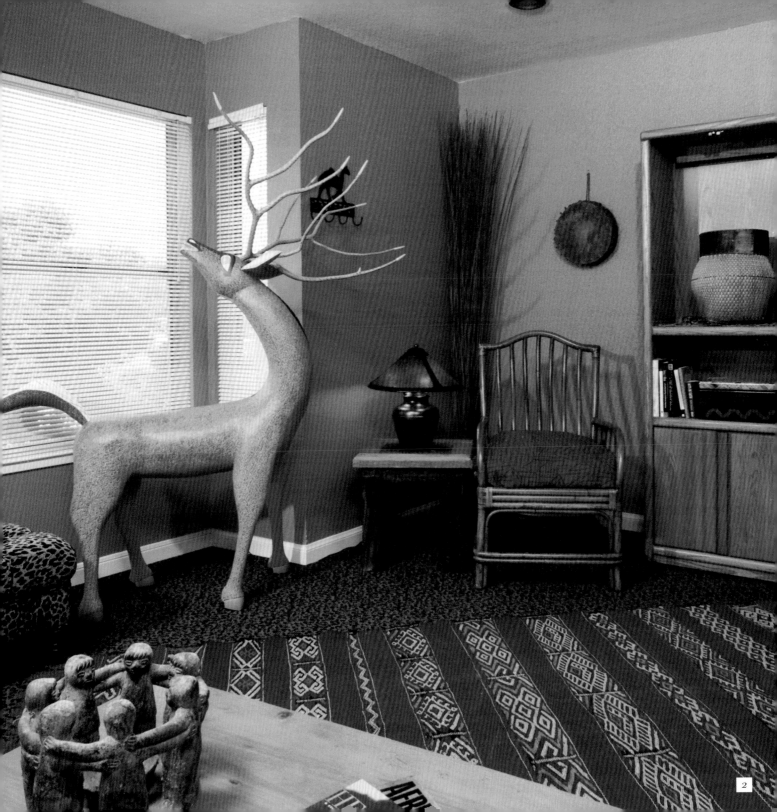

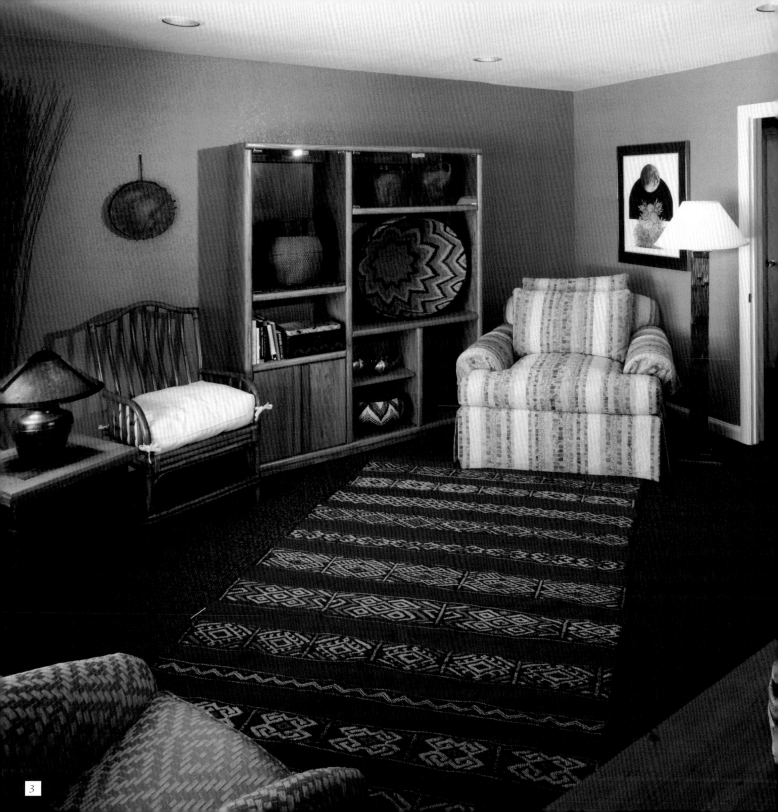

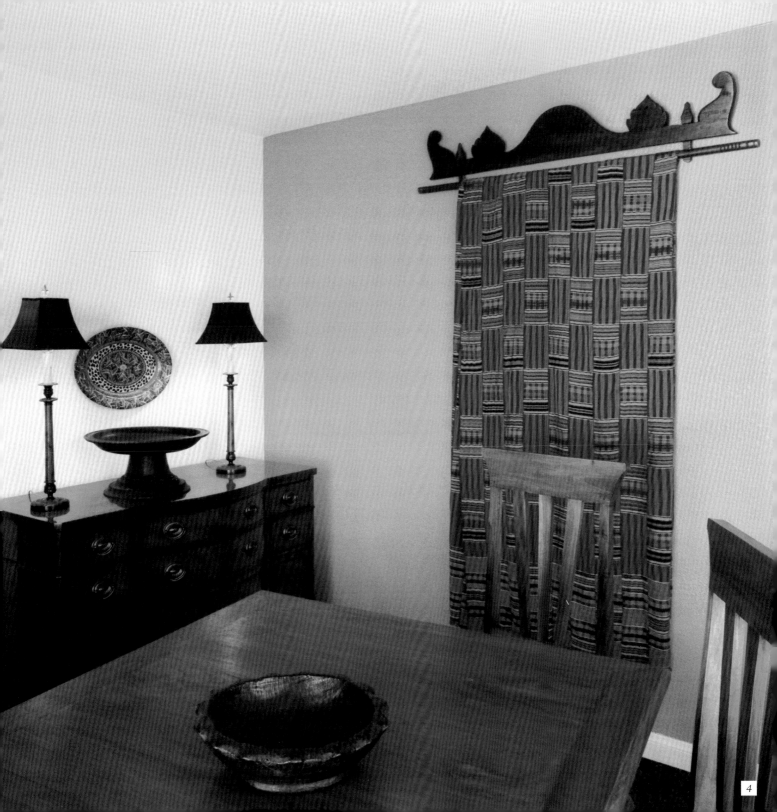

4

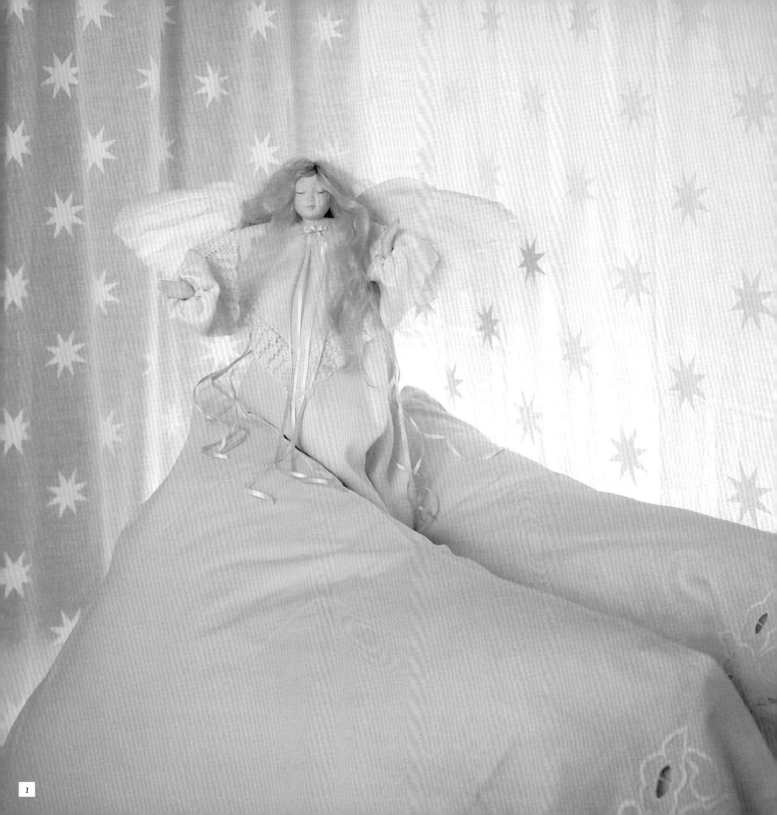

HEALING ENVIRONMENTS

Healing Environments

Healing Environments is a sanctuary for those who are suffering, a shrine for those who have suffered, and above all, a showcase for ways to relieve suffering. In August of 2003, Healing Environments moved from its Palo Alto location to a former antique store in one of San Francisco's loveliest neighborhoods. A resource center for the seriously ill and their caregivers, it includes extensive book, video and audiotape libraries and poetic spaces for remembrance and meditation, as well as a Jungian sandtray room. Headquarters for a small non-profit, Healing Environments is dedicated to the relief of suffering through the transformative power of beauty, art and meaning.

IMAGE INDEX:

Palo Alto Location: 1. Angel 2. Bedroom 3. Bedroom 4. Library 5. Gallery
San Francisco Location: 6. Sandtray 7. Sculpture 8. Resource Room

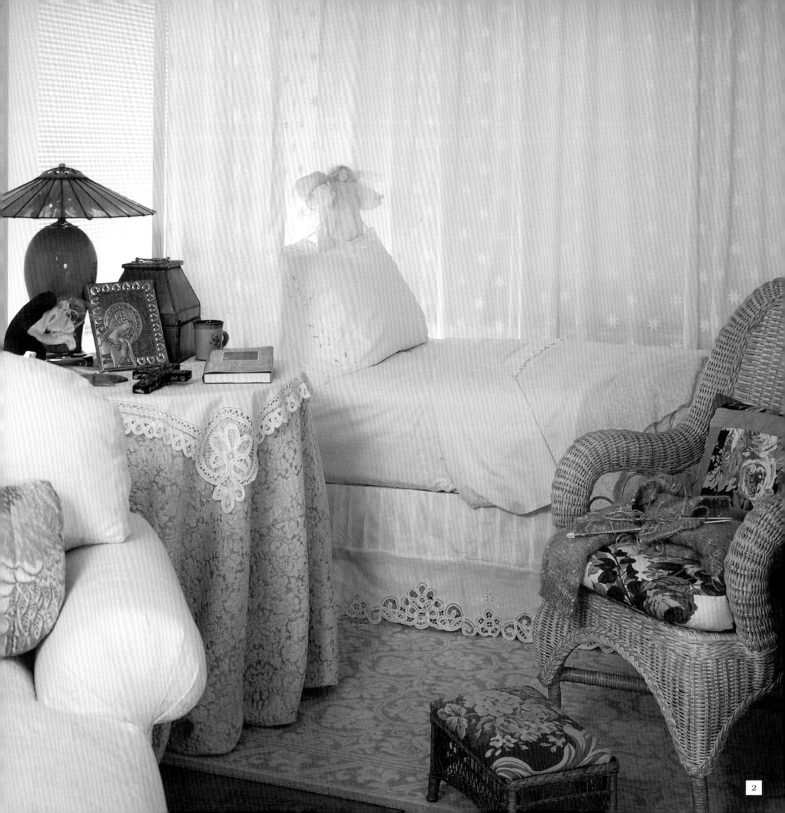

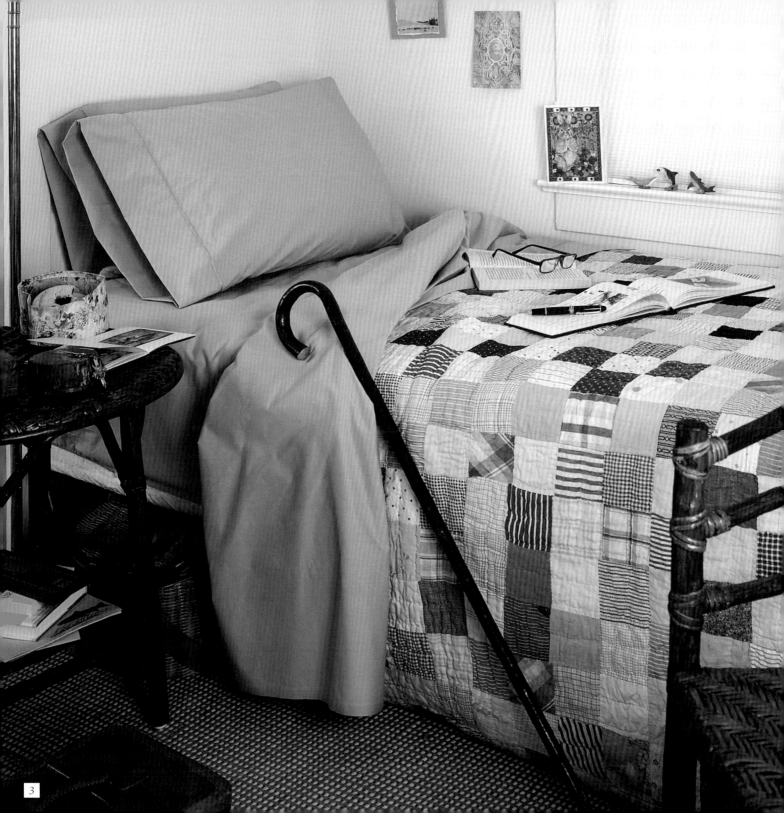

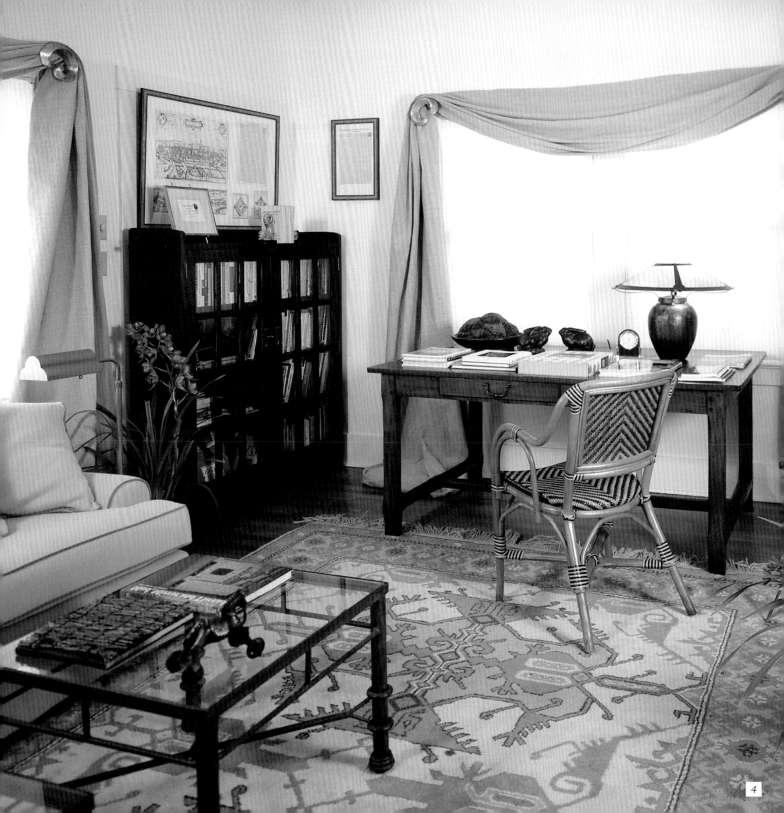

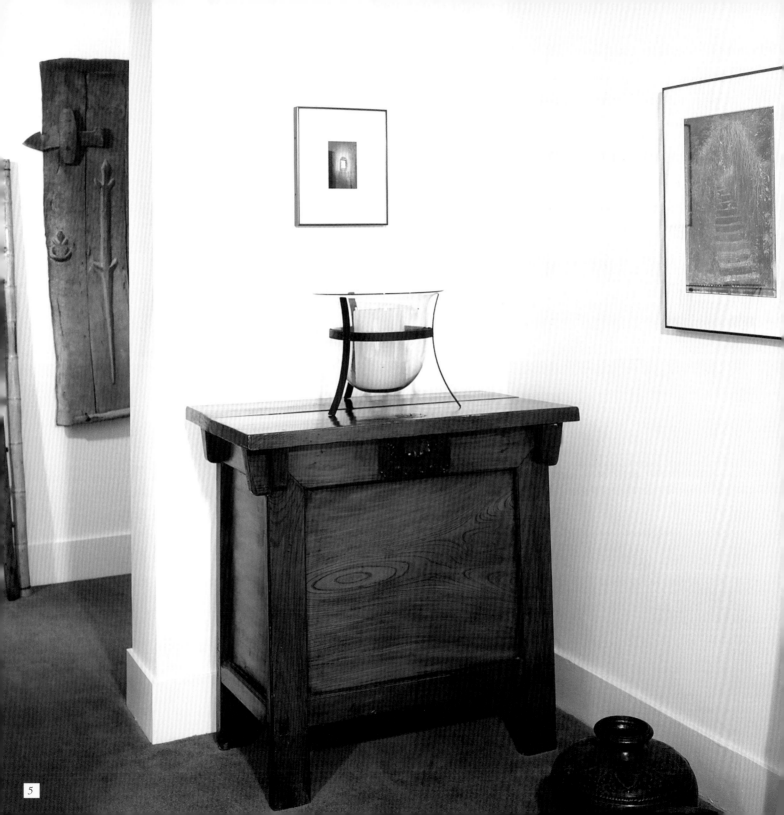

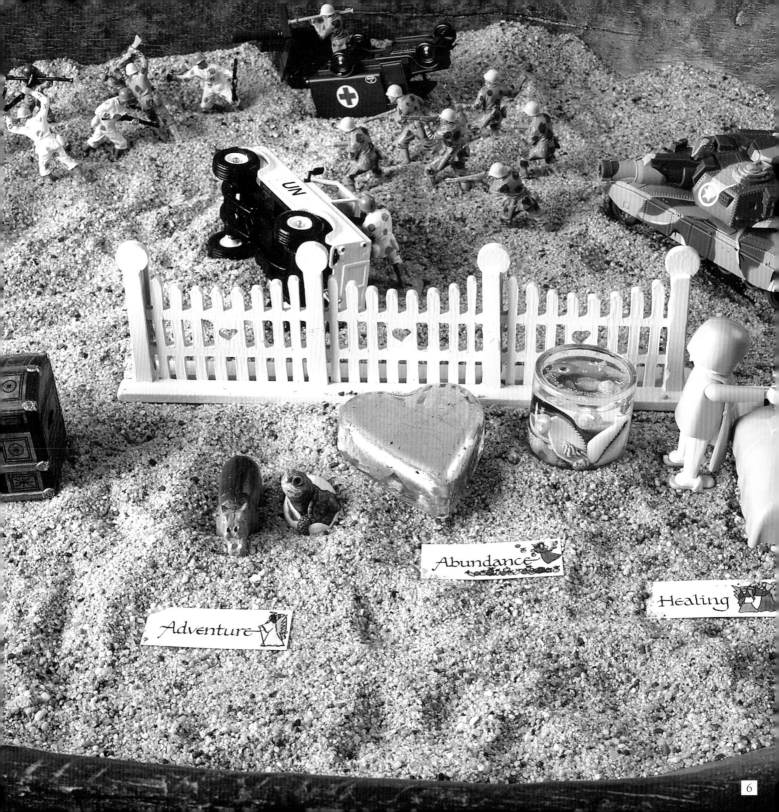

Adventure

Abundance

Healing

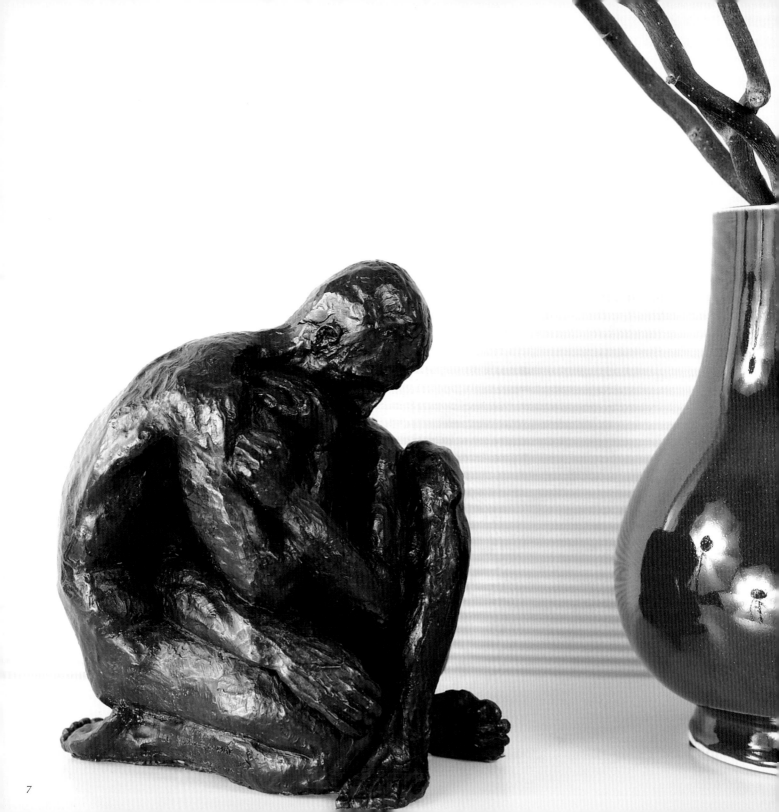

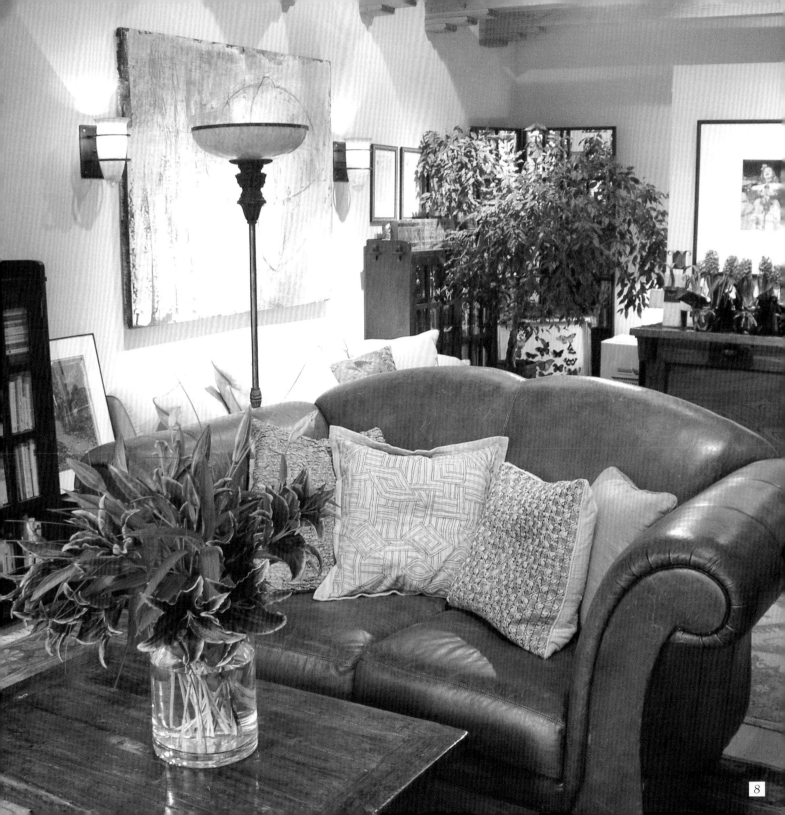

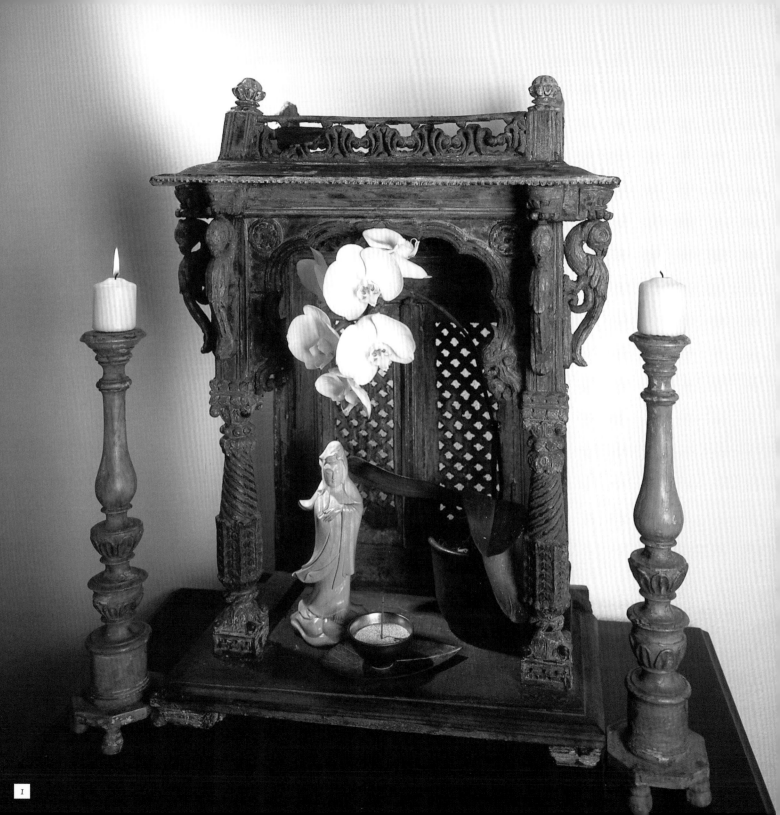

I

Healing Home
Palo Alto, California

Healing Home
Palo Alto, California

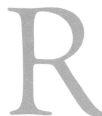esponding to requests that the design concepts of Healing Environments be applied to a home setting, codirectors Kate Strasburg and Traci Teraoka created this model for a Healing Environments fundraiser. In its four warm rooms, the two women sought to express their design philosophy with the rich layers of meaning offered by antiques, ethnic art, handcrafted objects, icons and nature itself.

IMAGE INDEX:

1. Altar 2. Living Room 3. Dining Room 4. Bedroom 5. Bedroom 6. Desk

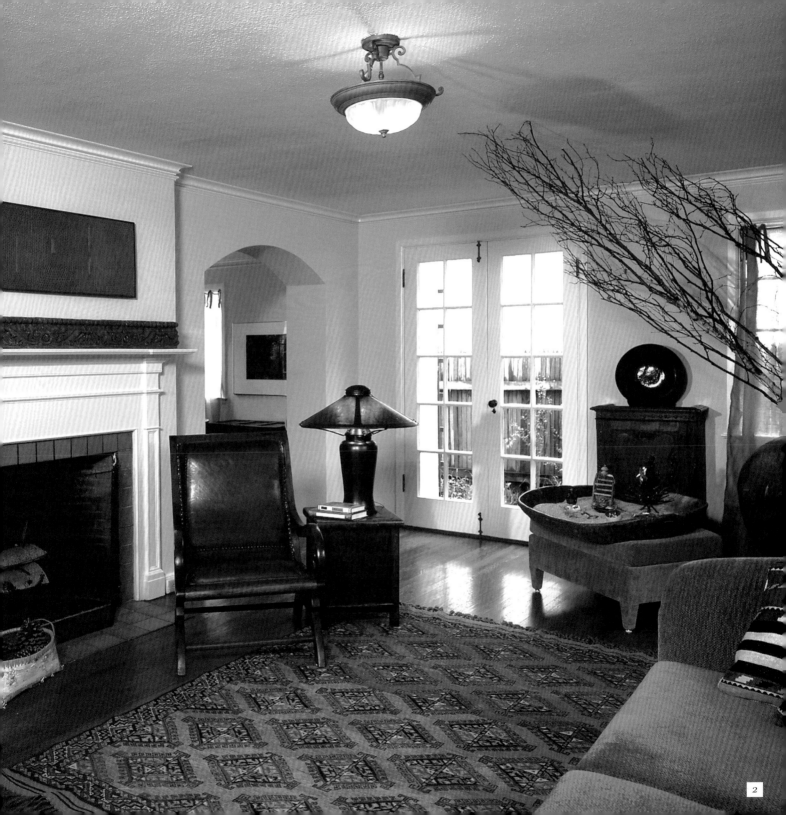

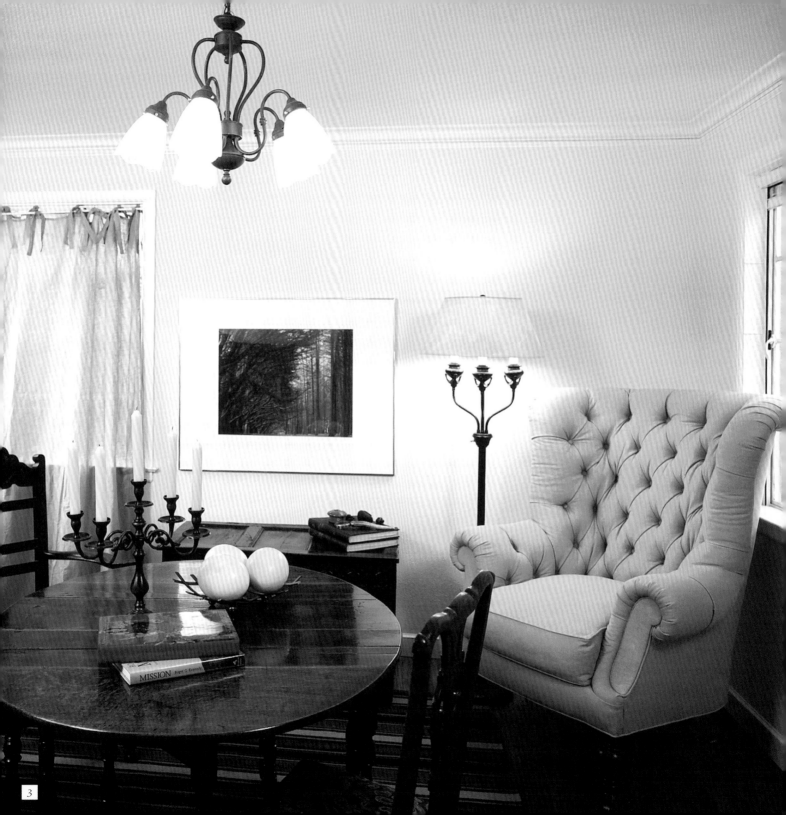

3

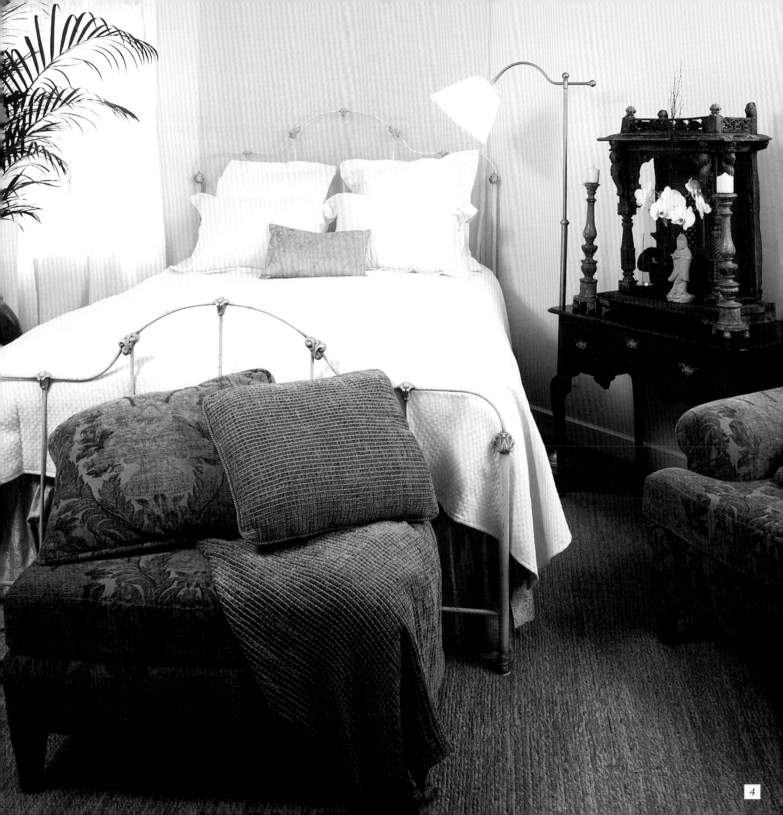

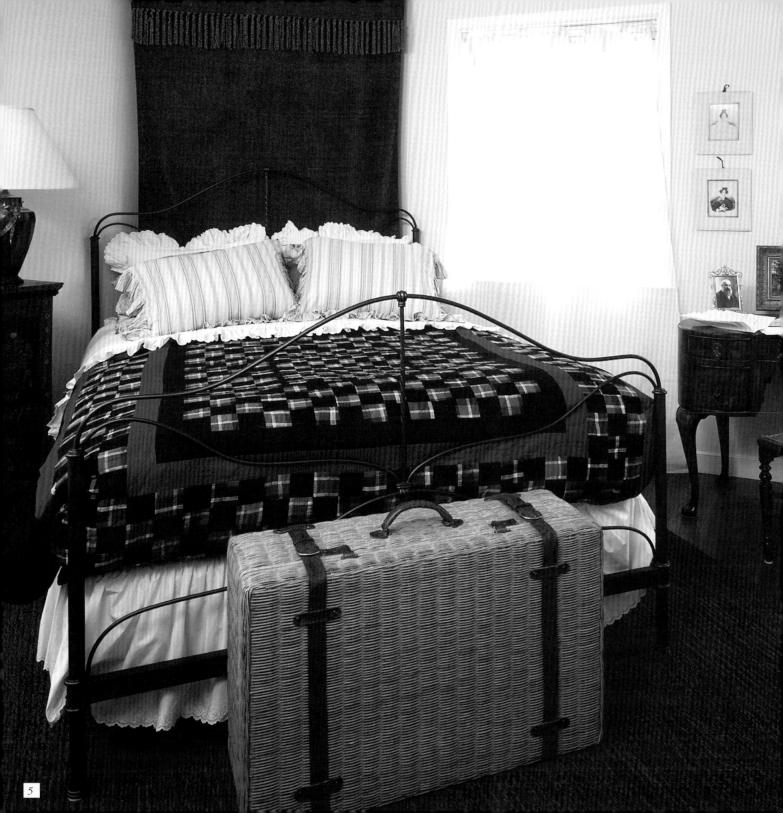

To those who have died alone

To those who have died well loved

To those who have died in pain

To those who have died in peace

To those who have died with lives fulfilled

To those who have died with dreams unlived

Healing Environments is dedicated

To the relief of all suffering

For we are one

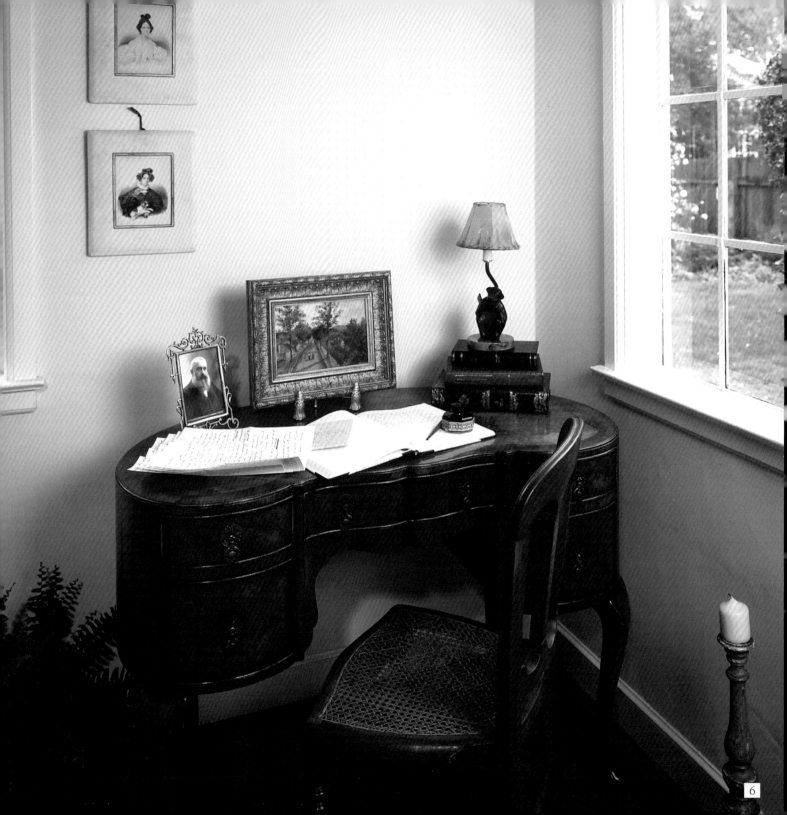

A DESIGN WORKBOOK

DEAR FRIENDS,

All of us need healing environments—whether patient or caregiver, healthy or ill. We need to align our physical environment with our deepest inner needs for optimal health and life satisfaction. We offer you this workbook as a tool for doing just that. Whether you wish to create a personal haven, support a loved one (or yourself) who is ill, or maximize the healing potential of your healthcare facility, use the guidelines and questions as starting points to launch you on your own journey of discovery. Think in terms of possibility—not limitations. Dare to dream and believe it can be done— you deserve it!

Kate / Traci

How
to Create a
Personal
Haven

START WITH INTENTION.

What are you seeking to accomplish? Do you hope to express your innermost self, honor a significant relationship, accommodate children, comfort one who is suffering? All of the above?

_____

_____

_____

_____

_____

_____

_____

_____

_____

_____

_____

_____

_____

ELIMINATE CLUTTER.

To create a sense of tranquility, limit the sensory input to a comfortable level.
Visitors to Healing Environments are always struck by its sense of peace,
but how to accommodate the chaos of life? Conceal it as much as possible.
Place it in closets or aesthetic containers: baskets, armoires, etc.

_____

_____

_____

_____

_____

_____

_____

_____

_____

_____

_____

_____

SURROUND YOURSELF WITH THINGS YOU LOVE.

When I moved into a small house after my divorce, my former husband said: "So this is what you wanted for twenty-three years!" A friend said that the rooms were so infused with who I was that it looked like a giant sandtray. If you surround yourself with things you love, your home will have a natural beauty and coherence. Consider including things with age, cultural artifacts, objects crafted by hand and heart, symbols with significance. Celebrate life and your own sense of identity. What well-loved things might you include in your ideal environment?

_____

_____

_____

_____

_____

_____

_____

_____

_____

_____

_____

_____

_____

HONOR YOUR PAST.

Sift through old letters and photographs to document your life. Frame a love letter. Surround a missing loved one's photo with flowers. Ancient cultures have always integrated the spiritual into the home. Create a shrine to honor your past and frame your future. How will you honor your past? How will you frame your future?

_____

_____

_____

_____

_____

_____

_____

_____

_____

_____

_____

_____

_____

_____

REVERE YOUR DREAMS.

Consider creating an "altar" on which to place a symbolic representation of what you wish in your life. At Healing Environments in Palo Alto we kept a current issue of our journal on the tatami mat in the meditation room. At home I keep a card with each child's name on my tiny chapel's altar. What will you place on your altar?

_____

_____

_____

_____

_____

_____

_____

_____

_____

_____

_____

_____

CREATE A RITUAL.

Frame your day. I check into my tiny closet chapel morning and evening. Monks in monasteries bless each time of day with prayer. Ritual can be used to transcend both time and distance. When my co-worker David and I were separated during my vacation, we maintained a sense of connection by meditating at the same time we had meditated together in Palo Alto: nine a.m. in California which was six p.m. in Greece. In pre-industrial times, man was grounded by his connection to the earth. In this age of computers and cell phones we must consciously struggle to maintain a sense of eternity amidst the pace of technology. With what ritual will you frame your day?

_____

_____

_____

_____

_____

_____

_____

_____

_____

_____

STRIVE FOR TRANSCENDENCE.

With whatever means possible, try to imbue your home with a physical representation of a higher or deeper level of reality. It is this which will sustain you through difficult times and ground you and your loved ones. How can you physically represent a higher or deeper level of reality?

_____

_____

_____

_____

_____

_____

_____

_____

_____

_____

_____

_____

_____

_____

INCLUDE MUSIC.

Find the music which best speaks to you and make it the background of your life. Use it, as Shakespeare once said, "to knit up the ravelled sleeve of care." Which music can best serve as background to your life? Which music speaks to you?

_____

_____

_____

_____

_____

_____

_____

_____

_____

_____

_____

_____

_____

_____

INCORPORATE NATURE.

Nothing speaks to one's place in the universe more than nature. Whether the serenity of a beautiful orchid, the joy of a canary's song, the lush growth of a fern, or the purring of a cat—nature, plant or animal, soothes us by placing us in the larger context of the natural world. How will you incorporate nature? Plants? Animals?

_____

_____

_____

_____

_____

_____

_____

_____

_____

_____

_____

_____

MAKE YOUR ART HEALING ART.

Select art which speaks to you and affirms your deepest longings. Art which reflects who you are. Art with meaning. Which pieces of art best reflect who you are?

_____

_____

_____

_____

_____

_____

_____

_____

_____

_____

_____

_____

_____

_____

BLESS YOUR HOME.

Bless yourself. You are a child of the universe. You deserve comfort, honor, reverence. Your life is sacred and deserves to be framed lovingly and with intention. You deserve a healing environment, a healing home, a haven. *Give thanks.*

_____

_____

_____

_____

_____

_____

_____

_____

_____

_____

_____

_____

_____

Additional Thoughts

_____

_____

_____

_____

_____

_____

_____

_____

_____

_____

_____

_____

_____

_____

_____

_____

_____

_____

GIVING FORM TO YOUR VISION:

SUPPORTING ONE WHO IS ILL

DESIGNING A HEALING ROOM

One November Traci and I were invited to address the Symposium on Healthcare Design in San Francisco. A great deal of good arose from this conference, but our favorite part of the presentation was an experiential exercise that we led. Our goal was to help our audience learn to design from "the inside out." By asking them to identify with a patient's deepest needs, we hoped to help them better address those needs.

We have included the exercise in this workbook in the hope that it may help other architects and designers as well as patients, their families and caregivers. Like all exercises which explore our deepest truths, it can only bring us closer to our most essential selves. And in sharing those truths it can only bring us closer to one another. For this exercise, imagine it is you who is seriously ill.

Haven

How can you make your room a haven? How can you effectively transform your surroundings to address your innermost needs? To nourish your soul?

_____

_____

_____

_____

_____

_____

_____

_____

_____

_____

_____

_____

_____

_____

COMFORT

How can you soothe each of your five senses?

What can offer soft textures to your touch? Flannel sheets? A mohair throw?

What colors will soothe your weary eyes? A sea-glass blue? A mushroom taupe?

What subtle scent will lull you to sweet dreams? Lavender?

What soothing sounds can calm your fragile nerves? A Bach cello suite?
A James Taylor song? The music of a small water fountain? The song of a bird?

What childhood favorite tastes can comfort your soul as well as nourish your body?
Custard? Bread pudding?

How can you imbue your surroundings with comfort?

_____

_____

_____

_____

_____

_____

_____

_____

_____

ORDER

What soothing sense of order will ground you?
How can you artistically conceal clutter?
Can you request flowers in your favorite combination
of colors and create an indoor garden?
Can reading materials be grouped in rattan baskets?
Can cards & photos be displayed on an artistic bulletin board?

_____

_____

_____

_____

_____

_____

_____

_____

_____

_____

_____

_____

EXPRESSION

What form of personal expression will energize you?
The more you express your individuality the more you are
empowered over your illness and institutional surroundings.
Can you wear special bedclothes?
Can you play your favorite music?
Can you display a favorite work of art?

_____

_____

_____

_____

_____

_____

_____

_____

_____

_____

_____

MEMORY

How can you expand time by infusing it with memory? Surround yourself with photos chronicling your life? Write your memoirs? Create a video to leave as a legacy?

_____

_____

_____

_____

_____

_____

_____

_____

_____

_____

_____

_____

_____

_____

MEANING

How can you expand time by infusing it with a sense of meaning?
How can you replace chronological time (*chronos*) with spiritual time (*kairos*)?
Remember the example of Viktor Frankl who said that even the horrors of a
concentration camp and death itself could not rob him of his wife's love.

_____

_____

_____

_____

_____

_____

_____

_____

_____

_____

_____

_____

Identity

How can you celebrate your life, your identity? What aspects of your identity can you express in your physical surroundings?

_____

_____

_____

_____

_____

_____

_____

_____

_____

_____

_____

_____

_____

_____

Icons

What personal icons or symbols can serve as touchstones?
Photos? Love letters? Religious or secular icons?

_____

_____

_____

_____

_____

_____

_____

_____

_____

_____

_____

_____

_____

_____

_____

RITUAL

What rituals can you create to overcome both time and distance, to transcend
the limitations your illness has placed on you?
Can you create a small altar? (In a suitcase if necessary!)
Can you pray or meditate at special times? Can you ask absent friends and family
to "sign up" for an hour of the day or night to send a healing thought or prayer
your way or to meditate or pray with you from a distance?
Can you counteract the institutional setting with transcendent music?

_____

_____

_____

_____

_____

_____

_____

_____

_____

_____

_____

ESSENCE

How can you use your physical surroundings to return you to your essence?
How can you infuse your personal surroundings with your essence so that you
effectively transcend the institution which threatens to subsume you?

_____

_____

_____

_____

_____

_____

_____

_____

_____

_____

_____

_____

_____

_____

_____

_____

_____

TRANSFORMATION

How can this illness become your key to transformation? How can you overcome the physical limitations which your illness places upon you and let your spirit soar?

_____

_____

_____

_____

_____

_____

_____

_____

_____

_____

_____

_____

_____

LIGHT

How can your illness lead you into the light? As Joseph Campbell said:
. . . at the bottom of the abyss comes the voice of salvation. The black moment is the moment when the real message of transformation is going to come. At the darkest moment comes the light.

_____

_____

_____

_____

_____

_____

_____

_____

_____

_____

_____

_____

_____

_____

ADDITIONAL THOUGHTS

IN YOUR HEALTHCARE SETTING,
DO YOU HAVE A HEALING ENVIRONMENT?

RATE THE FOLLOWING SPECIFIC AREAS IN TERMS OF THEIR PATIENT-CENTEREDNESS:

(on a scale of 1 to 10)

1. ER	1 2 3 4 5 6 7 8 9 10	6. Signage	1 2 3 4 5 6 7 8 9 10
2. Waiting Rooms	1 2 3 4 5 6 7 8 9 10	7. Gift Shop	1 2 3 4 5 6 7 8 9 10
3. Patient Rooms	1 2 3 4 5 6 7 8 9 10	8. Food Service	1 2 3 4 5 6 7 8 9 10
4. Treatment Rooms	1 2 3 4 5 6 7 8 9 10	9. Garden	1 2 3 4 5 6 7 8 9 10
5. Hallways	1 2 3 4 5 6 7 8 9 10	10. Chapel	1 2 3 4 5 6 7 8 9 10

_____

_____

_____

_____

_____

_____

_____

_____

_____

_____

THOUGHTS & IDEAS

WHAT IN YOUR PHYSICAL ENVIRONMENT...

1. Puts patients at ease? Makes them feel welcome? (*Addresses fear and discomfort.*)

_____

_____

2. Meets individual needs and concerns?

_____

_____

3. Treats the patient with dignity and respect? (*Validates her thoughts and feelings? Makes him feel like more than a diagnosis?*)

_____

_____

4. Meets emotional needs? (*Gives a sense of caring and comfort.*) Meets spiritual needs? (*Gives hope and a sense of transcendence.*)

_____

_____

5. Instills trust and confidence? (*Once again overcoming fear.*)

_____

_____

Thoughts & Ideas

WHAT IN YOUR HUMAN ENVIRONMENT...

1. Puts patients at ease? Makes them feel welcome? (*Addresses fear and discomfort.*)

_____

_____

2. Meets individual needs and concerns?

_____

_____

3. Treats the patient with dignity and respect? (*Validates her thoughts and feelings? Makes him feel like more than a diagnosis?*)

_____

_____

4. Meets emotional needs? (*Gives a sense of caring and comfort.*) Meets spiritual needs? (*Gives hope and a sense of transcendence.*)

_____

_____

5. Instills trust and confidence? (*Once again overcoming fear.*)

_____

_____

For Families

1. What overcomes fear?

_____

_____

_____

2. What improves communication?

_____

_____

_____

3. What guarantees comfort?

_____

_____

_____

4. What addresses grief and loss?

_____

_____

_____

THOUGHTS & IDEAS

For Staff

1. What empowers them?

_____

_____

_____

2. What improves communication?

_____

_____

_____

3. What nurtures them?

_____

_____

_____

4. What addresses grief and loss?

_____

_____

_____

WHAT ARE THE TEN BEST THINGS ABOUT YOUR HEALTHCARE SETTING?

1) _____

_____

2) _____

_____

3) _____

_____

4) _____

_____

5) _____

_____

6) _____

_____

7) _____

_____

8) _____

_____

9) _____

_____

10) _____

_____

WHAT ARE THE TEN WORST THINGS ABOUT YOUR HEALTHCARE SETTING?

1) _____

_____

2) _____

_____

3) _____

_____

4) _____

_____

5) _____

_____

6) _____

_____

7) _____

_____

8) _____

_____

9) _____

_____

10) _____

_____

THOUGHTS & IDEAS

WHAT TEN THINGS WOULD YOUR IDEAL HEALTHCARE SETTING CONTAIN?

Physical Environment

1) _____

_____

2) _____

_____

3) _____

_____

4) _____

_____

5) _____

_____

6) _____

_____

7) _____

_____

8) _____

_____

9) _____

_____

10) _____

_____

THOUGHTS & IDEAS

WHAT TEN THINGS WOULD YOUR IDEAL HEALTHCARE SETTING CONTAIN?

Emotional Environment

1) _____

_____

2) _____

_____

3) _____

_____

4) _____

_____

5) _____

_____

6) _____

_____

7) _____

_____

8) _____

_____

9) _____

_____

10) _____

_____

THOUGHTS & IDEAS

THOUGHTS & IDEAS

THOUGHTS & IDEAS

To those who have died alone

To those who have died well loved

To those who have died in pain

To those who have died in peace

To those who have died with lives fulfilled

To those who have died with dreams unlived

Healing Environments is dedicated

To the relief of all suffering

For we are one